CW00835591

SIMPLE DIAGNOSTIC TESTS

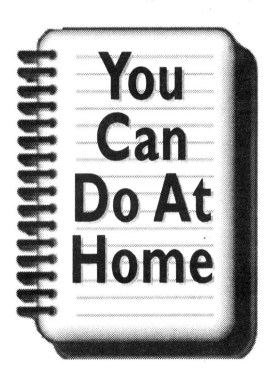

You Can Do At Home

by Martha M. Christy

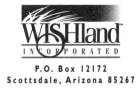

WISHland
INCORPORATED

P.O. Box 12172
Scottsdale, Arizona 85267

Simple Diagnostic Tests
You Can Do at Home

by Martha M. Christy

ISBN 0-96332091-3-2
EAN 9 7809633209138
First Printing — June, 1995
Second Printing — August, 1998
Copyright © 1995 Martha M. Christy All Rights Reserved.

Printed in the United States of America.

TABLE OF CONTENTS

INTRODUCTION

I n the last half of our century, huge increases in population and the allure of high-profit assembly line medicine has placed an enormous strain on the quality of health care no matter where you live. Hurried, impersonal and expensive doctors visits are unpleasant and too often don't provide the needed time and care to ensure proper diagnosis and treatment.

That's why so many of us today are turning to self-medical care at home. When we care for ourselves and for our family members' health, we can take more time, in a more relaxed atmosphere, to carefully consider what's ailing us and what our symptoms mean.

Even doctors themselves are encouraging us to learn more about our own health because the more prepared and knowledgeable we are, the more we can help our health care providers quickly and efficiently determine what illness we may be experiencing and what to do about it.

All of us naturally turn to self-diagnosis and treatment when we feel sick. We eliminate rich foods when we have an upset stomach; we rest more and drink more fluids when we have colds, we take our temperature or touch our forehead and skin to determine if we have a fever.

These are all simple, natural ways of diagnosing and treating our illnesses at home. But there are many more simple tests that you can perform right at home to monitor your health and to detect illness or disease right at home. And several of these tests are the very same tests that your doctor or health practitioner performs when you make an office visit.

In *Simple Diagnostic Tests You Can Do At Home*, we're going to look at some of the excellent home testing methods that are available to you today. Tests like urine observations and urine dipstick testing are very simple to do and very accurate. As a matter of fact, statistics are now showing that in many cases home testing can be MORE accurate than screening tests done in a doctor's office or lab.

And it makes sense. At home, you're more relaxed, and you're taking the test under normal circumstances in a familiar atmosphere (no rushing to make an office appointment, less anxiety about test results, no dodging crowds and hurried receptionists in the waiting room).

So let's learn more about how you can monitor your health at home as often as you want, for hundreds of dollars less, and in a relaxed and caring environment with simple diagnostics tests you can do at home!

CHAPTER ONE:
URINE TESTING

The Best and Simplest Home Tests

When you make a visit to the doctor's office what's one of the first things the nurse asks you to do? She gives you a small cup and asks you to give her a urine sample—right? Well, have you ever stopped to think what's so important about your urine samples and why the doctor or hospital asks for them so often?

IN THIS CHAPTER

■ How Urine is Formed

Actually, what most people don't realize is that urine is actually filtered blood, and so contains nearly all the same constituents that your blood contains. For this reason, your urine sample can often tell as much about the condition of your health as a blood test. But a urine sample is a lot simpler, less expensive and definitely much less painful than a blood test, so urine tests are the often the first diagnostic tool that the doctor turns to when you have symptoms of illness.

Because urine tests are so simple and convenient and tell so much about the state of your health, there have been many, many thousands of research studies on how to use urine to detect illnesses or abnormalities in the body. As one very prominent urinalysis researcher stated:

"Urine has been referred to as a mirror which reflects the activities within the individual's body...urine provides information about the functions of the whole body."

—— **A.H. Free (Former president of Miles Laboratories)**

So now you can begin to see why urine testing is so important--it tells so much about your body and your health and yet it's so simple and easy to do, that urine testing can even be done at home.

A well-known doctor of internal medicine says that:

> *"When it comes to the simplest, relatively least expensive way to monitor one's personal health especially to detect some oncoming or latent disease urinalysis probably offers more generalized health information than any other home test...yet the information that you can obtain can be as valuable as that provided by the most sophisticated professional laboratory."*
>
> —— **Dr. Edward Pinckney, Do-It-Yourself Medical Testing**

Today, home urine testing is becoming one of the most popular self-help tools available. It's simple, inexpensive, very accurate and so saves a whole lot of time and money on doctor's visits and blood tests. Home pregnancy urine tests for instance, provide tremendous freedom, convenience and almost instant results, without the trouble, bother and expense of doctor visits and blood testing.

Home urine testing can also help you to help your doctor make an early diagnosis of an illness or disease before it gets out of control. When you detect an abnormality during home testing, you can bring it to your doctor's attention so that he can take further steps if necessary. This type of preventive medicine helps you to take control over your own health and to become an active participant in your own health care

For those of you who use natural healing methods at home, urine testing can also show you what progress you're making with your natural medicines. For instance, if you suddenly develop burning on urination, you can test for a bladder or urinary tract infection with a simple urine dipstick. If the test is positive, you can then use the natural remedy of your choice such as an herb or a homeopathic medicine such as Cantharis.

After using the treatment a few times, you can retest yourself with the urine dipstick to see if the test is now negative at which time you would taper off or stop your natural treatment.

Before we get into the self-testing tools and procedures, let's look first at what urine is and how it's formed in the body, because knowing a little basic anatomy will give you a clearer idea of why the analysis or testing of urine is so important.

HOW URINE IS FORMED IN THE BODY

Many people believe that urine is formed in the intestines as a by-product of digestion, but this is not true. In reality, urine is made by KIDNEYS, not the digestive tract. Actually, urine, because it is part of the circulatory system, never passes through the digestive tract at all and is never mixed with the solid wastes that are excreted from the body through the colon.

This is the way that urine is made in the body:

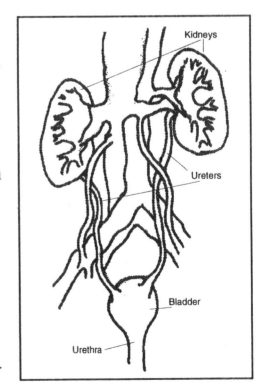

Female Urinary System

1 The blood that flows through your capillaries, veins and arteries is chock full of hundreds of different elements—nutrients, water, enzymes, hormones, salts, minerals, white and red blood cells, antibodies and many, many other complex elements which govern and regulate the functions of the whole body.

2 The body has to continually regulate the amount of each and every element in the blood so that there is never too much or too little of water, salt, calcium, hormones, antibodies, red and white blood cells, etc., in the system which would cause an imbalance in the body's functioning.

11

3 The organs that are primarily responsible for balancing the amount of these elements in the blood are the KIDNEYS. Without the kidneys, the blood levels of salt, water, hormones, etc. would become too high or too low and the body would be unable to function. (You can see why kidney damage or disease can be so devastating or even fatal).

4 As the blood enters the kidneys, it's absorbed into a long, very complex system of intricate tubes called nephron (this is where the word nephrologist, which means a kidney specialist, comes from). There are about 1.25 million nephrons in each kidney and within each nephron are tiny filtering capillaries called glomeruli which continually absorb and filter the blood.

5 The glomeruli sift, sort, filter and re-filter the elements in the blood, reabsorbing many elements and excreting small amounts of substances that the body doesn't need at the time. For instance, if you've had a lot of salty meals one day, the glomeruli will filter out and excrete the excess salt from the blood through the bladder, so that your serum (blood) salt levels are normalized.

6 As the blood is selectively filtered again and again in the glomeruli, it gradually becomes what is called a 'plasma ultrafiltrate' which basically means a very

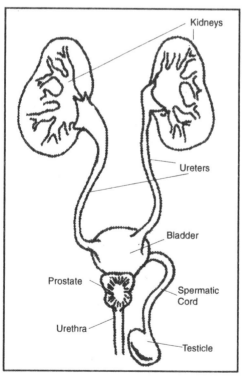

Male Urinary System

pure, filtered form of blood. This ultrafiltrate is actually what we call urine.

7 Much of the ultra-filtered blood, or urine, is reabsorbed back into the bloodstream, in order to renourish the blood. Any excess urine that is not presently needed by the body at the time is excreted by the kidneys. The urine flows down through two small tubes connected to the kidney called ureters. The ureters carry the urine to the bladder.

8 Once the urine is ready to be excreted from the body, it flows down a tube connected to the bladder called the URETHRA, and out of the body.

Because the urine contains almost every element found in the blood, it provides an excellent source for testing what's going on in the body. Disease or illness causes changes in blood chemistry. And because urine is essentially filtered blood, these changes in blood chemistry can in many cases be detected through the urine.

Urine testing today is highly accurate and because urine tests are painless and simple to perform, they provide an ideal way to regularly monitor and test yourself for a wide variety of possible health abnormalities.

In the next two chapters we're going to look at two different types of urine testing:

 Appearance of the urine

The appearance of your urine——its color, clarity, volume and odor of are actually very important health indicators and observing all of these regularly is an excellent home testing regimen. Testing your urine for appearance doesn't require any special preparation or tools and can be done at any time.

2 Prepackaged urine dipsticks

Certain pharmaceutical companies make and sell plastic dipsticks to which one or more small styrofoam-like pads are attached. The pads change color if there is something abnormal in the urine such as blood or protein.

These dipstick are simple and easy to use and can test for many different conditions. When using urine dipsticks, it's best to collect the urine specimen by means of a 'clean catch'. We'll talk about how to do that later on in the section on dipstick testing.

Both of these methods of urine testing have high rates of accuracy when performed correctly, and are excellent tools for your personal preventive and diagnostic home care.

CHAPTER TWO:
THE APPEARANCE OF URINE
What It Can Tell About Your Health

Most people don't realize just how much the appearance of your urine can tell you about what's going on in your body. Observing certain things about your urine can be extremely important clues to uncovering health abnormalities that you may not be aware of and will also help you to practice preventive care by revealing the presence of conditions that are just beginning.

There are lots of things that can temporarily change the normal appearance of your urine such as certain foods, drugs or excessive exercise. Occasional temporary changes in the normal appearance of your urine don't necessarily mean that you have a health problem, but repeated patterns of abnormalities such as continually cloudy or very dark urine, unusually frequent and heavy urination, etc. can be very accurate warning signals of illness or disease.

So let's see how to test for abnormalities in urine appearance and learn how to interpret early warning signs of problems in the body.

IN THIS CHAPTER

■ **How to Test Urine Appearance**

■ **Urine Color**

■ **Urine Odor**

■ **Urine Clarity**

■ **The Three Glass Test**

■ **Urine Volume**

THE URINE APPEARANCE TESTS:

These are five simple, basic urine observations that can tell you a host of things about your health: color, odor, clarity (cloudy or clear), volume, and frequency of urination).

> **Urine Appearance**
> 1. Color
> 2. Odor
> 3. Clarity (cloudy or clear)
> 4. Volume
> 5. Frequency of urination

Testing your urine appearance frequently is an excellent way to discover undiagnosed health conditions. Also, using these urine self-testing methods can help you to determine how well a treatment you're using is working.

Observe your urine before and after treatment to determine if urine abnormalities disappear following the treatments. If they fail to improve after several days, it may indicate that the treatment you're using is not working effectively.

HOW TO TEST URINE APPEARANCE

TOOLS YOU'LL NEED:
When testing the appearance of your urine use a clean, clear glass container (preferably 16 oz.). The container doesn't have to be sterile but make sure that the container has been thoroughly washed in hot water and rinsed well so that it's free from soap and other residues.

COLLECTING THE SAMPLE:
Urinate normally into the container (collect all that

you pass)). Then set the container on a level surface in normal light (out of bright sunlight or bright artificial lighting). You can test urine appearance at any time of the day. Just follow the directions in next few pages which tell you how to interpret the appearance of your urine.

WHEN SHOULD I TEST:
It's a good idea to observe your urine color, odor, clarity, volume and frequency regularly (at least 3-4 times a week).

If you are ill or suspect that you may have an undiagnosed condition, observe your urine every time you urinate for 2-3 days.

Observe what patterns repeatedly emerge and compare them with the charts and information in this chapter.

You can also follow up your appearance test with dipstick tests (see next chapter) for confirming the urine appearance tests. When abnormal appearances are observed, especially if they occur repeatedly, contact your doctor for follow-up testing.

Now we're going to look at each individual factor of urine appearance in detail so that you can learn to detect health problems simply by observing your urine.

I. URINE COLOR

Urine color can be an important indicator of illness or disease. This is because the color of urine often changes during many disease states due to the presence of pigments produced during illness that don't normally appear in the urine.

For example, pigments from abnormal liver bile may produce a yellow-brown or greenish color; other pigments from liver substances may produce an abnormal brown urine color; abnormal hemoglobin in urine gives a reddish brown-color and so on.

Let's see how urine color can reveal many different types of health problems.

WHAT'S NORMAL?

Morning Urine: NORMALLY APPEARS A MEDIUM TO DARK AMBER color, because you are not eating and drinking at night, so your urine becomes very concentrated with minerals, salts, etc. which gives it a darker color.

Afternoon and Evening Urine: Afternoon and evening urine: NORMALLY BECOMES LIGHT YELLOW (LIKE STRAW) as you begin diluting the urine by eating and drinking during the day.

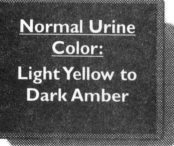

Normal Urine Color:

Light Yellow to Dark Amber

The yellow or amber color of normal urine is due to a yellow pigment called urochrome which is present in the urine.

ACCURACY OF URINE COLOR TESTING

An abnormal change in urine color is considered to be 90 percent accurate as an indication of some dysfunction in the body (as long as the color change is not due to normal causes such as drugs, foods or exercise).

HOW TO TEST URINE FOR COLOR

You can test for urine color any time you pass urine. Just remember that your urine is normally darker amber in the morning and becomes lighter yellow after eating and drinking fluids through the day.

Abnormal urine colors are explained in the following pages. Read over each page so that you have some idea of what each abnormal urine color can indicate.

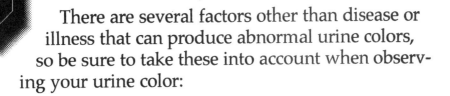

BEFORE YOU TEST, CONSIDER THIS:

There are several factors other than disease or illness that can produce abnormal urine colors, so be sure to take these into account when observing your urine color:

DRUGS:

Before doing the color test, if you are taking medication, first check the drug labeling or ask your doctor if the drug affects the urine color. That way, you'll know that any abnormal urine color is probably due to the drug and not to a health problem. If your urine color is different from what the drug is supposed to produce, check back with your doctor, especially if the urine color is a black.

FOODS:
Natural food coloring (such as beets) or food dyes can affect the color of your urine, so make sure that you consider what you've been eating when testing urine color.

 DEHYDRATION:
- **Vigorous exercise**
- **Sweating**
- **Vomiting during illness:**

Urine can appear a darker amber or more vivid yellow color under these conditions because there is less water in the urine, so the solids (salts, minerals, etc.) are more concentrated, making the urine appear darker amber or a more vivid yellow color than usual. Be sure to take all of these factors into account when observing your urine color.

INTERPRETING URINE COLORS

WHAT'S NORMAL?

Light yellow to dark amber are normal urine colors.

WHAT'S NOT NORMAL?

Abnormal urine colors are:

- Pink
- Red/Orange
- Brown
- Yellow/Orange
- Blue/Green
- Black

- Red
- Peach
- Vivid Yellow
- Green
- Very Dark (Brown)
- White (clear)

Color Chart I

Pink, Red or Brown Color Shades

COLORS	MAY INDICATE	MOST COMMON CAUSES
Pink to Red Red-orange Peach Brown	Blood in urine (from kidney stones, urinary tract infections) Liver disease	Foods: beets, rhubarb, berries Food dyes or coloring Laxatives: Ex-Lax, Senekot, etc. Drugs: Pyridium, Mellaril and others (check with your doctor Menstruation

**Pink, Red, Red-Orange, Peach, Brown Urine Colors
may indicate:**

BLOOD IN THE URINE:

Most often indicates a urinary tract infection. Infections such as cystitis, bladder infections and kidney infections can produce blood in the urine.

LIVER DYSFUNCTION:

Porphyrins are naturally occurring iron/magnesium substances found in the body. However, liver dysfunction may produce abnormally large amounts of porphyrins in the bloodstream and urine, changing urine color to a red-orange, pink, brown or red color.

WHAT TO DO:

If your urine color is any one of the colors in the chart above, make sure that you have considered all the most common causes of these color changes first. If none of them applies, follow up the color test with the urine dipstick tests for **Blood, Bilirubin and Urobilinogen** (see next chapter). If your urine color or dipstick test for urine in the blood are positive, report your findings to your health practitioner immediately.

Report any abnormal test results (color or dipstick or both) immediately to your health practitioner.

Color Chart II

Vivid Yellow to Yellow Orange

COLORS	MAY INDICATE	MOST COMMON CAUSES
Vivid Yellow	Anemia	Dehydration
Vivid Yellow-Orange	Thyroid Disease	Foods (carrots)
	Decreased kidney function	Drugs: sulfa drugs, laxatives or others

Vivid Yellow to Yellow Orange may indicate:

ANEMIA OR THYROID DISEASE:
A continually repeated pattern of vivid yellow or yellow-orange urine color may indicate severe anemia or a problem with the thyroid.

KIDNEY DYSFUNCTION:
A vivid yellow or yellow-orange urine color that is seen repeatedly and is not due to one or more of the common causes listed above, is often a sign of a problem with the kidney.

WHAT TO DO:

If your urine is **repeatedly** a vivid yellow to yellow/orange color and none of the most common causes listed above apply, use the urine dipstick tests for **Blood**, **Protein** and **Leukocytes** to see if any abnormalities appear (see next chapter). Even if the urine dipstick tests mentioned are negative, report any abnormal chronic yellow - yellow orange urine color to your health practitioner..

Unfortunately, diagnostic tests for early or subliminal kidney disease are not particularly accurate. If you cannot confirm a diagnosis, but your urine is continually vivid-yellow or yellow-orange, and you have accompanying symptoms of burning and pain on urination, you may find the help you need by contacting a homeopathic doctor and describing your symptoms.

Homeopathic medicine is prescribed on the basis of symptoms, rather than on often ineffective technical diagnostic testes. Homeopathic remedies such as Berberis or Cantharis are well-known to ease kidney stress and urinary tract problems, and offer safe, effective relief from kidney and other urinary tract infections.

Parsley, dandelion root tea and marshmallow tea also have been traditionally used to strengthen and cleanse the kidneys and urinary tract.

Color Chart III

Green to Blue-Green

COLORS	MAY INDICATE	MOST COMMON CAUSES
Green	Bacterial infection	Foods or food dyes
Blue-Green	Liver or Galbladder problems	Drugs: Indocin, Elavil

Greenish or Blue-Green Urine Color may indicate:

LIVER DYSFUNCTION
GALL BLADDER PROBLEM
GENERALIZED BACTERIAL INFECTION

Some types of liver dysfunction or systemic bacterial infections may cause urine color to change to a shade of green or bluish green.

 ## WHAT TO DO

If you observe a green to blue-green urine color, first make sure that none of the most common causes listed above apply. Follow-up the color test with a urine dipstick test for **BILIRUBIN AND UROBILINOGEN** (see next chapter).

These two dipstick tests are used primarily for detecting liver dysfunction, but can also detect certain types of generalized infections in the body such as mononucleosis that harm blood cells.

If either or both the color and dipstick tests show abnormalities, contact your doctor for further testing.

Color Chart IV

Black or Dark Brown

COLORS	MAY INDICATE	MOST COMMON CAUSES
Black Brown	Melanin in the urine (a pigment of skin cancer) Old blood from the bladder	Naphthalene (moth repellent) poisoning

Black or extremely dark urine may indicate:

SKIN OR OTHER CANCER
URINARY TRACT INFECTION OR DISEASE
CHEMICAL POISONING

Black urine is an extremely abnormal health sign. Contact your health practitioner at once if you observe this urine color at any time.

 WHAT TO DO

If your urine color is black or nearly black at any time, follow-up immediately with a multistix 10 dipstick screening test (see next chapter) and then report your findings to your doctor immediately.

Color Chart IV

Clear to White

COLORS	MAY INDICATE	MOST COMMON CAUSES
Very Clear	Early sign of diabetes	Excessive Water Intake
White	Kidney dysfunction	

Clear to White Urine Color may indicate:

KIDNEY DYSFUNCTION:
When the kidneys are not functioning properly, they may not excrete normal amounts of excess solids (salts, proteins, etc.) into the urine. This makes the urine appear very clear, or almost white.

DIABETES:
One of the earliest signs of diabetes the passing of extremely large amounts of very clear, watery urine, due to hormone imbalances.

WHAT TO DO

If your urine is consistently very clear or colorless over a period of several days, and if you're also passing a very large amount each time you urinate, it could be an early sign of diabetes. Check the section on **Urine Volume** in this chapter and the section on **Glucose Dipstick Testing** in Chapter 3.

Extended Color Test

Leave a urine sample standing for 1-2 hours after observing the original color. In some cases, the urine will darken to red-brown or black when particular metabolic or inherited health conditions such as arthritis are present. Consult with your doctor if this test is positive.

II. URINE ODOR

For many centuries, the scent or odor of urine was observed in making medical diagnoses for such things as diabetes (sweet odor), or urinary tract infections (ammonia odor). Even today, some doctors will ask their patients to eat a strong-smelling food such as asparagus in order to see how long it takes before the odor is detectable in the person's urine.

If the odor is detectable soon after eating, it can indicate that the kidneys are not filtering as efficiently as they should be, which can indicate a possible kidney infection or an early sign of kidney disease.

ACCURACY:
Abnormal urine odor is about 60% accurate in indicating a health problem.

WHAT'S NORMAL?

Urine should normally have very little odor. The typical smell of urine is believed to be due to the presence of certain proteins and metabolic acids. Old urine, or urine that is left standing without refrigeration will take on the odor of ammonia because of the decomposition of urea (the primary salt in urine).

WHAT'S NOT NORMAL?

Sweet or Fruity Odor: Can indicate a problem in carbohydrate metabolism as in Diabetes. In this disorder, due to faulty metabolism of starches and fats, the body produces an over-abundance of acids called ketones which produce a sweet or fruit-like odor in the urine. But this odor can also be present in those who are fasting or dieting and eating none or very few carbohydrates. This process of increased ketone production due to abnormal carbohydrate metabolism is called ketosis. Your dip-stick urine tests (see next chapter) will confirm the presence of abnormal ketone levels.

Maple Syrup Odor: In infants, this odor can indicate an inherited disorder called 'maple syrup disease', in which the enzyme necessary for breaking down certain amino acids (lysine, leucine or isoleucine)is missing. Treatment usually includes a diet which avoids these proteins or in rare cases, transfusions or dialysis (mechanical cleaning of the blood).

Disagreeable Odor: A strong, ammonia-like or unusually strong smell that is not due to food may be an indication of an impending or present urinary tract infection. A urine dipstick test (see next Chapter) for Nitrites (acid salts) and Leukocytes (white blood cells) will confirm if you have a urinary tract infection such as a bladder or kidney infection

'Foul' Odor: An unusually bad urine odor that is not due to food is sometimes present in diseases such as cancer.

In observing urine odor, remember that you're looking for a pattern, in other words, abnormal odors that occur consistently or continually.

III. URINE CLARITY

Urine should be a clear, even sparkling light yellow especially immediately after urinating; (after standing, urine can appear cloudy, but this is normal).

ACCURACY:
Cloudy urine is considered to be about 75% accurate in indicating a health problem, although it does not point to a specific condition. A follow-up check with urine dipsticks tests should be done when you see that your urine is cloudy. The dipsticks will confirm the presence of abnormal bacteria, proteins, salts, etc. in your urine.

WHAT'S NORMAL?

Normal urine is clear, sparkling yellow and free of floating deposits.

WHAT'S NOT NORMAL?

Cloudy urine is not normal urine. Milky, or cloudy urine contains substances that should not be present such as bacteria, proteins, phosphates (phosphoric salts), fats or vaginal discharges in women. An exception to this is the fact that a man's urine may appear cloudy after sexual activity. Urine that is very alkaline can also be cloudy. Abnormally alkaline or cloudy urine can be caused by urinary tract infections or kidney dysfunction.

Continually Cloudy Urine May Indicate

Most Commonly	Very Occasionally
Kidney stones (early warning) or kidney dysfunction	Diabetes
	Sexually transmitted disease
Bladder infection or infection elsewhere in the urinary tract	Lymph system problem
	Possible tumor at some location in the body

WHAT TO DO

When your urine is consistently cloudy (each time you urinate for 2-3 days), it's always best to use a full-screen urine dipstick test which will confirm the presence of abnormal salts (Nitrites), protein (kidney problem), Leukocytes (white blood cells that indicate infection), and other elements. Read the instructions in the next chapter on full-screen urine dipstick testing, and check to see if you have any positive test results.

THE THREE GLASS TEST FOR CLOUDY URINE:

If your urine appears to be consistently cloudy and you want to try to pinpoint where the infection is occurring in the urinary tract, the three-glass test can help.

HOW TO DO THE 3-GLASS TEST:

1 Gather together 3 clean, clear glass containers (no soap or detergent residue).

2 When you first get up in the morning, pass a small quantity of urine into the first glass, then the midstream urine into the second glass, and the last small portion of urine into the third glass.

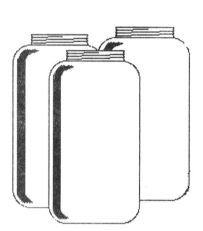

3 Place the three glasses side by side on a level surface and observe.

WHAT THE THREE GLASS TEST CAN INDICATE:

■ If all three glasses of urine are clear, then your test results are normal.

■ If the small amount of urine in the first glass is cloudy, but the second glass is less cloudy, it usually indicates an infection in the urethra (the tube leading from the bladder to the opening where the urine leaves the body). One fairly common cause of urethral infections is sexually transmitted diseases.

■ If the first container is clear and the second glass is cloudy, it may indicate a bladder or kidney infection.

■ If both the first and second glasses are cloudy, a urinary tract infection is indicated.

■ If the urine in the third glass is cloudy, it can indicate a bladder infection that is just beginning or, in men, a possible prostate problem.

ACCURACY:
The Three-Glass Test is considered to be 80% accurate in helping to pinpoint where a urinary tract infection is located and is especially good for detecting the presence of sexually transmitted diseases such as chlamydia or gonorrhea.

IV. URINE VOLUME

The amount of urine you pass changes everyday in response to the amount of water you drink and types of foods eaten. However, there are certain guidelines as to how much or how little urine is normally passed. Consistent or extreme deviations from normal urine volume can be one of the first important indicators of disease.

NORMAL THINGS THAT AFFECT URINE VOLUME:

■ Decreased urine output for women just prior to menstruation is normal.

■ Increased fluid intake during exercise normally increases urine volume.

■ Cold weather can increase urine volume because less water is lost through perspiration. Warm weather decreases urine output because the body is conserving water.

■ Diuretics and some medications increase or change urine output (check with your doctor).

TAKING THE TEST:

Collect all of the urine you pass in one 24-hour period in a large wide-mouth one or two quart container. After all urine is collected, measure total urine quantity in a measuring cup or container with ounce markings.

WHAT'S NORMAL?

One to two quarts of urine passed per day is normal for the average person on a typical diet.

Be sure you have first considered all of the normal factors that can influence urine output (listed on page 32) when evaluating your Urine Volume Test.

WHAT'S NOT NORMAL?

Urine OutPut Greater Than 2 Quarts per Day May Indicate:

- *Diabetes mellitus:* a form of diabetes caused by improper metabolism of carbohydrates due to a chronic insufficiency of insulin (often called sugar diabetes).

- *Diabetes insipidus:* a form of diabetes caused by insufficient secretion of the anti-diuretic hormone (ADH). ADH prevents excessive loss of water by the body. In diabetes insipidus, too much water is excreted in the urine, causing severe dehydration and extremely elevated salt levels in the body. (Often referred to as water diabetes).

- *Kidney Disease:* In some forms of kidney disease, the kidney tubules do not respond to the anti-diuretic hormone (ADH) and too much water is excreted from the body, causing a form of diabetes insipidus.

- **Kidney Stones**

- **Metabolic Disorder**
- **Kidney stones in the bladder** (frequent urination during the day, but not at night)

Urine OutPut less Than 1-2 Quarts per Day May Indicate:

- Kidney Disease
- Heart Disease
- A urinary tract obstruction
- An intestinal obstruction
- A hormone imbalance
- A severe emotional reaction

WHAT TO DO

Report all clearly abnormal changes in urine volume to your doctor. Urine output of less than 8 oz. in a 24 hour period should be considered a medical emergency.

As you can see, simply observing certain characteristics of your urine can tell you a lot about what's going on in your body and can even alert you to serious illness or disease.

In the next chapter, we're going to look at how you can follow up urine observations with urine dipstick testing at home.

Urine dipstick tests give you fast accurate, professional results that not only save you time and money, but also help you monitor your health regularly.

CHAPTER THREE
URINE DIPSTICK TESTS
Professional Diagnostic Tests You Can Do At Home

Urine dipstick tests offer more general information about your whole health picture than just about any other home test you can use. And the fact that they're so simple to use and inexpensive, makes them an ideal way to monitor some of our most important body functions without continual, expensive and stress-causing doctor's visits.

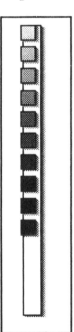

Multistix

Urine dipsticks are simply plastic strips to which one or more small styrofoam-like pads have been attached. Each pad on the dipstick has been treated with what is called a "reagent". A reagent (usually a clear liquid) is simply a chemical that will change color in the presence of some other substance. For instance, white blood cells in your urine that are produced during a urinary tract infection will make a particular reagent change color. If there is no infection and no white blood cells, the reagent does not change color.

On the urine testing dipsticks, different specific reagents have been added to the small pads that are affixed to the plastic strips. Dip the strip in your urine and voila! The pads will change color if there is something abnormal in your urine such as blood, sugar, abnormal proteins, etc.

IN THIS CHAPTER
■ Types of Dipstick Tests
■ Getting Ready for Testing
■ Clean Catch Samples
■ Multistix Tests
● Leukocytes
● Nitrites
● Urobilinogen
● Protein
● pH
● Blood
● Specific Gravity
● Ketone
● Bilirubin
● Glucose

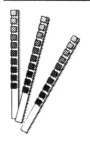

Doctors use urine dipstick tests extensively, but they also are sold for home use. Unfortunately, one of the biggest problems with urine dipstick tests for home use is that most people do not understand the medical terminology that's commonly used in the directions for interpreting the results of urine dipstick testing. Terms like bilirubin, specific gravity or urobilinogen can make your eyes cross. But don't despair. In this chapter, we're going to go through each urine dipstick test step-by-step and explain how each one works and how to interpret the test results in language that's simple to understand. So let's get started!

WHAT TYPES OF URINE DIPSTICK TESTS ARE AVAILABLE?

First of all, let's go over what urine dipstick tests you can buy for home use. There are several separate urine dipsticks available for separate tests such as the bladder infection, or urinary tract urine test, the kidney infection urine test, etc. But one of the most cost-effective and comprehensive urine testing methods you can buy are what are called the urine Multistix tests.

The urine Multistix dipsticks contain several different pads for multiple urine tests on one dipstick. Some Multistix contain six pads for six different tests, while other brands contain up to 10 pads on one dipstick for performing 10 different and very important medical tests.

In this chapter, we're going to use the Miles (or Ames) Multistix 10 dipsticks as our guide. There are other brands of Multistix available, but this particular brand is widely distributed and considered to be excellent quality.

By learning to use the Multistix urine tests, you can gain a broader understanding of what health problems you can detect through performing the same 10 basic and most common urine tests that doctors themselves perform.

GETTING READY FOR DIPSTICK TESTING

The Clean Catch Sample

For dipstick testing, a urine sample is obtained by means of a 'clean catch'. A 'clean catch' urine sample is done so that you can to eliminate factors that might falsely influence the outcome of your urine dipstick tests, such as bacteria on the exterior genitalia. Such bacteria might possibly contaminate your urine sample and produce a false positive test result such as mistakenly indicating a bladder infection, for instance. So it's important to clean the exterior area around the area where the urine passes out of the body.

Also, during menstruation, any blood on the outer genitalia could be picked up in a 'non- clean catch' urine sample, and so your urine test would show blood in the urine, but this would not be an indication of a health problem.

A clean catch urine specimen also includes collecting the midstream urine only, because this also helps to eliminate factors that may mistakenly affect the outcome of the urine tests.

For women's directions on how to do a 'clean-catch', see the directions on page 37. 'Clean catch' directions for men are on page 38.

HOW TO DO A 'CLEAN CATCH' FOR WOMEN:

1. Soak a clean washcloth in warm, soapy water and wring out lightly.

2. Spread the outer lips of the vaginal opening and wash from FRONT TO BACK with warm soapy water. DO NOT wash from back (anal area) to front, as this can spread contaminating bacteria from the colon to the vaginal area.

3. Rinse the washcloth with hot water and wash the vaginal area again with clear warm water (from front to back). Pat dry with a piece of sterile cotton.

4. To collect the urine, spread the outer vaginal lips, pass a small amount of urine into the toilet and begin collecting the 'midstream portion' of the urine only. Pass the last small portion of the urine into the toilet.

5. Those of you who have done 'clean catches' at the doctor's or gynecologist's office know that the nurse gives you a package with a sterile cup and antiseptic wipes for the clean catch. You can use antiseptic wipes that are sold at the drugstore if you want, but the warm, soapy water is just as effective and is more natural.

6. Also, if you don't have a sterile cup on hand, just make sure that the one you use has been washed in very hot, soapy water and has been well rinsed in clear, hot water so that it is really clean and free of soap or other residue.

7. A glass cup or container is preferable for urine testing so that you can also observe the appearance of the urine which can indicate many different health conditions.

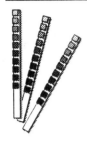

WHEN TO TEST

In general, you can use the urine dipstick tests by collecting a urine specimen at any time of the day.

For some of the dipstick tests (such as Specific Gravity and pH), you'll be looking for repeated patterns and so more frequent testing throughout the day may be indicated.

You'll find more information on the best time for testing in the information given for each specific test further on in this chapter.

HOW TO DO A 'CLEAN CATCH' FOR MEN:

1. Retract the foreskin of the penis, then wash the tip of th penis with warm soapy water. Rinse and pat dry with a piece of sterile cotton.

2. Discard the first small portion of urine, collect the midstream urine in a clean glass and discard the last small portion of the urine stream.

3. Those of you who have done 'clean catches' at the doctor's office know that the nurse gives you a package with a sterile cup and antiseptic wipes for doing the clean catch. You can use antiseptic wipes that are sold at the drugstore if you want, but the warm, soapy water is just as effective and is more natural.

4. Also, if you don't have a sterile cup on hand, just make sure that the one you use has been washed in very hot, soapy water and has been well rinsed in clear, hot water so that it is really clean and free of soap or other residue.

5. A glass cup or container is preferable for urine testing so that you can observe the appearance of the urine which can indicate many different health conditions.

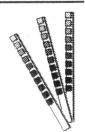

GETTING TO KNOW THE MULTISTIX 10 URINE SCREENING TEST

The Multistix 10 Reagent Strips for Urinalysis (urine dipsticks) are thin, white plastic strips and come packaged with an accompanying color chart (either on a separate sheet or attached to the bottle itself).

On the color chart you'll see several long horizontal columns containing the name of the test and various blocks of color.

Take your finger and point to each column on the color chart. On the far left of each column you'll see the following words in bold (these are the specific names of each urine test on the Multistix 10):

1. **LEUKOCYTES**
2. **NITRITES**
3. **UROBILINOGEN**
4. **PROTEIN**
5. **PH**
6. **BLOOD**
7. **SPECIFIC GRAVITY**
8. **KETONE**
9. **BILIRUBIN**
10. **GLUCOSE**

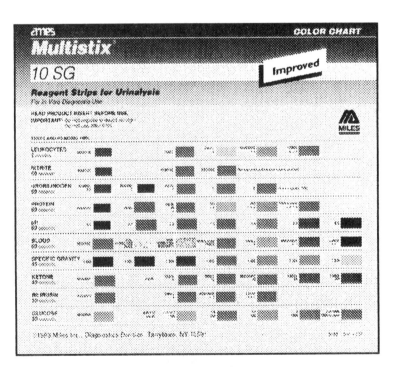

Multistix Color Chart

The terms in the list above are unfamiliar to most of us, so before we get started on the directions for taking the Multistix dipstick test, let's get familiar with what each of these 10 tests mean so that you can interpret your test results without confusion.

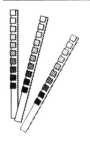

I'm going to go through each of the 10 tests named above in detail so that you'll know exactly what they mean and how to use them.

I. LEUKOCYTES

In the Leukocyte test, you'll be testing for a possible urinary tract infection. A leukocyte is actually a particular type of white blood cell that your body normally produces to fight an infection or inflammation. When an infection or inflammation occurs in the urinary tract, the numbers of leukocytes (or white blood cells) increase. At this point, the increased number of leukocytes can usually be detected in your urine by taking the simple Leukocyte urine dipstick test.

The urinary tract includes the kidneys, ureters (tubes that carry urine from the kidney into the bladder), the bladder, the urethra (tube that drains urine from the bladder to the outside of the body), and the prostate in men (see illustration on page 12).

Urinary tract infections are very common—-a reported 30 million women and some 1 million men have symptoms each year. Common symptoms are burning, and sharp pains or discomfort when urinating. Undiagnosed urinary tract infections can lead to chronic inflammation, pain, burning and discomfort on urination and to possible kidney disease or prostate problems, so it's important to make sure that you take the Leukocyte test periodically, especially if such symptoms are appearing.

The Leukocyte test is extremely accurate (90% accuracy) and is the primary test performed in doctor's offices, hospitals and labs for detecting urinary tract infections.

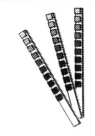

BEST TIME FOR TESTING

The first urination in the morning when you get up is usually the recommended time for testing.

BEFORE YOU TEST, CONSIDER THIS:

INTERPRETING THE TEST

Make sure that you wait 2 minutes from the time you dip the stick in the urine to read the Leukocyte test result.

NORMAL: After dipping, the Leukocyte test pad will match the ivory color (Negative) color block.

ABNORMAL: If the Leukocyte dipstick pad (the top pad on the stick) matches any other color block in the LEUKOCYTE column on the color chart (darker beige to purple) your Leukocyte test is positive and indicates a possible:

- Bladder infection
- Infection in the urethra or ureters
- Kidney infection

WHAT TO DO IF YOUR TEST IS POSITIVE

1 If your Leukocyte test is positive, report the results to your health practitioner.

2 Also check the NITRITE, PROTEIN and BLOOD tests on the dipstick carefully, as these are added indicators of uri-

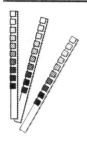

nary tract infections. Report all positive test results to your health practitioner immediately.

3 The Leukocyte test indicates the presence of a urinary tract infection, but it doesn't pinpoint where the infection is located. You can use the Three-Glass urine test on page 31 to help determine where the infection is located in the urinary tract..

4 Traditional herbal treatments for urinary tract infections include: marshmallow tea (one quart per day until symptoms are relieved), red clover tea, parsley tea, dandelion root, uva ursi, goldenrod tea and nettle.

Traditional, very effective homeopathic treatments include: Berberis (3 granules 3 per day) and Cantharis 3 granules 3 per day).

5 To determine how your treatments are working (this includes conventional treatments), take the Leukocyte test 1-2 days after starting the treatment. You'll see that the test pad will change to its normal color (tan) as the infection improves or is alleviated). This is an excellent, inexpensive method for monitoring your urinary tract infection and the success of your treatment methods at home.

II. THE NITRITE TEST

The urine Nitrite dipstick test is commonly used by doctors to detect bladder infections or an infection elsewhere in the urinary tract. During a urinary tract infection, bacteria present in the urine (while it's being stored in the bladder) changes certain types of dietary salts called nitrates to another form of salt called

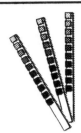

nitrites. The Nitrite dipstick test will detect the abnormal nitrite salts in the urine, which can indicate a urinary tract infection.

However, just because your nitrite test is negative, it doesn't necessarily mean that you don't have a urinary tract infection, because not all types of bacteria present during a urinary tract infection will change nitrates to nitrites in your urine. So make certain, particularly if you have symptoms of a urinary tract infection (burning and pain on urination), that you check the Leukocyte test pad, as well as the Nitrite test pad for color changes.

BEST TIME FOR TESTING

The first morning urine catch is best for Nitrite testing

BEFORE YOU TEST, CONSIDER THIS:

■ The urine to be tested should have been in the bladder at least four hours before testing.

■ Use only fresh urine for testing. After standing 30 minutes, the urine sample can produce a false-positive test.

■ Large amounts of Vitamin C intake can cause a false-negative test result. Stop taking Vitamin C supplements at least 24 hours before testing.

■ Urine with a high specific gravity (see page 57) may cause a false-negative test result.

■ Certain drugs that color the urine red can cause a false-negative nitrite test.

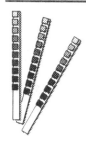

INTERPRETING THE TEST

NORMAL: The Nitrite test pad remains white (Negative).

ABNORMAL: If your Nitrite test is positive, the test pad will turn pink. Any shade of pink indicates a positive test result (the presence of a urinary tract infection).

IF YOUR TEST IS POSITIVE

1 If your Nitrite test is positive, check the Leukocyte test pad, the Blood test pad and the Protein test pad also. All of these tests can confirm the Nitrite test and can indicate inflammation or infection somewhere in the urinary tract that is either just starting or is progressing.

2 For treating urinary tract infections, see the treatment suggestions in the Leukocyte section.

III. UROBILINOGEN

Urobilinogen is one of the many end products of the process of the normal breakdown of red blood cells in the body. When old red blood cells die after their normal lifespan (about four months), the hemoglobin contained in the cells is released and then broken down into bilirubin (the orange-yellow pigment that colors liver bile). Later, urobilinogen is formed in the intestines from the bilirubin. Urobilinogen is absorbed into the liver and is excreted from the body through both the urine and in solid waste.

Abnormal amounts of Urobilinogen which can be detected in the urine dipstick test most commonly signal liver or bile duct

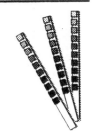

disease. This is because the liver is not absorbing urobilinogen properly and consequently, abnormal amounts of urobilinogen show up in the urine.

BEST TIME FOR TESTING

The Urobilinogen test can be performed in the morning using your first morning sample.

BEFORE YOU TEST, CONSIDER THIS:

■ Your urine test sample must be no more than 5 minutes old.

■ The pH of your urine sample should be somewhere around 5.0 to 7.5. Very acid urine (5.0 and below) may produce a false negative result. Overly alkaline urine (over 7.5) can produce a false positive result. You can check your pH with separate pH test papers before the Urobilinogen test.

■ Drugs may produce inaccurate results (check with your doctor or pharmacist to determine whether any medication you may be taking will interfere with this test).

INTERPRETING THE TEST

NORMAL: Your urine dipstick Urobilinogen pad should match the peach (or Normal) color blocks on the color chart.

ABNORMAL: **Decreased Urobilinogen**: If the color on your Urobilinogen test pad does not match ANY of the color blocks in the Urobilinogen column on the color chart, it may indicate an abnormal

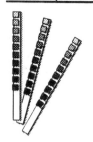

ABSENCE OR DECREASE in urobilinogen which may be caused by:

- Liver or bile duct obstruction
- Infection or inflammation of the bile ducts
- A tumor or growth which is obstructing the bile ducts
- Antibiotic therapy which is suppressing normal intestinal flora and preventing conversion of bilirubin to urobilinogen

Excess Urobilinogen: Small amounts of urobilinogen are normally present in the urine, but larger amounts of it in the urine indicate that red blood cells may be breaking down at an abnormal rate. The raspberry colored blocks to the right in the Urobilinogen column on the color chart indicate a positive test for excess Urobilinogen in the urine.

A positive test result for excess Urobilinogen can indicate:

- Different types of anemia.
- Malaria
- Infectious hepatitis
- Cirrhosis
- Congestive heart failure
- Infections such as mononucleosis

IF THE TEST IS POSITIVE

 If your Urobilinogen test is positive, check the Bilirubin test pad on the dipstick for results. The bilirubin test can often help distinguish liver disease from a problem with the red blood cells themselves.

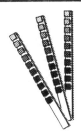

 Report all abnormal urobilinogen test results immediately to your health practitioner.

IV. PROTEIN

Your blood contains microscopic proteins called albumins and globulins. The albumins attach themselves to hormones, enzymes and even vitamins and drugs and carry these elements throughout the body. Globulins help transport immune substances to where they are needed in the body.

As your blood flows through the kidneys most of these proteins are returned to the bloodstream, and only extremely minute amounts are filtered from the blood and end up in the urine. But if there are particular dysfunctions in the body, such as kidney disease, heart disease, diabetes, infections, or cancer, the amount of protein in the urine can increase and can be detected through a simple urine dipstick test.

 BEST TIME FOR TESTING

The Protein test may be performed at any time during the day.

 BEFORE YOU TEST, CONSIDER THIS:

■ Vigorous exercise, prolonged standing, chilling, certain antibiotics and some sleeping medicines can cause a false-positive protein test result. Test again after eliminating any of these conditions that apply to you. Your second test should be negative once these factors have been eliminated.

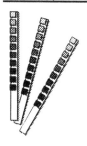

■ Your urine should not contain detectable protein. If your first test is positive, test again and if the second test is positive, report the results to your doctor.

■ Most doctors discount an occasional trace amount of protein in the urine, but if you see a continuing pattern of trace protein each time you test, report it to your doctor. Also, if your Protein test is positive, make sure you check the Leukocyte and Blood test pads, as a positive result from these can indicate that the protein in your urine may be caused by damage to the kidney caused by inflammation, infection or obstruction.

INTERPRETING YOUR TEST RESULTS

NORMAL: If the Protein test pad matches the pale yellow (Negative) color block in the Protein column on your color chart, your test is is normal or negative.

ABNORMAL: Abnormal protein levels in the urine are indicated by color changes from light green to aqua on the Protein test pad which indicate possible:

■ Kidney disease or infection
■ Other urinary tract disorders such as a bladder infection
■ Certain forms of heart and artery disease
■ High blood pressure
■ Diabetes
■ Hormone imbalances
■ Infections at any location in the body
■ Different forms of cancer
■ Sexually transmitted diseases
■ Rare conditions such as lupus or amyloidoisis (abnormal protein deposits in tissues and organs often connected with diseases such as

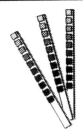

tuberculosis, osteomyelitis, rheumatoid
arthritis or Crohn's disease).
- Liver, nerve or thyroid dysfunction
- Viral diseases
- Possible metal or chemical poisoning

IF THE TEST IS POSITIVE

1 If you get an abnormal Protein test result, retest yourself
again 4-6 hours later. Then repeat the test for 2-3 succes-
sive days. If you get abnormal test results everyday, or a
majority of days, report the results to your doctor for evaluation. The doctor will refer to abnormal protein in the
urine as proteinuria or albuminuria.

2 Check the BLOOD and LEUKOCYTE test pads carefully.
These tests can help the doctor pinpoint what may be con-
tributing to the protein in your urine. These tests also can
indicate problems such as kidney infections, kidney
stones, etc., that can cause kidney dysfunction and result
in abnormal protein levels in the urine. Report all positive
tests to your doctor immediately.

V. pH

pH means 'potential hydrogen' and refers to your body's ability
to take in and utilize hydrogen atoms, which directly affects
how acid or alkaline your body fluids, cells and tissues are.

This is critically important because everything in your body
including your blood, cells, intracellular fluids, even your skin
and hair cannot be maintained in healthy condition without the
proper pH balance. A continuing pattern of abnormal urine pH

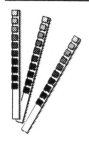

can indicate the onset or progress of many different diseases, so pH testing is very important.

For frequent pH testing, it's cheaper and more precise to use separate pH papers (see order form in back), but the Multistix give you the advantage of noting if your pH reading is accompanied by other abnormal readings. For instance, the combination of an acid pH and an abnormal Glucose test could indicate possible diabetes; an acid pH plus an abnormal Protein test might indicate a possible kidney problem and so on.

BEST TIME FOR TESTING

The pH test can be performed at any time during the day (see below for more instructions).

BEFORE YOU TEST CONSIDER THIS:

■ To measure pH, we refer to numerical values. Acid/alkaline levels in the body usually range from 4.5 (very acid) all the way up to 8.0 (very alkaline).

When you get up in the morning, your urine pH should normally be rather acid (4.5 - 5.5). As you eat and drink through the day, your body should become more alkaline—— 6.0 - 7.0 by midday and 7.0 - 8.0 by evening. This fluctuation in pH from 4.5 to 8.0 during the day is normal.

■. Many different things will alter your pH. Acid foods such as large quantities of meats, fish, dairy products or poultry products can acidify your system and produce highly acid urine. Grains such as rice, millet and barley have a more alkaline effect on the body, while vegetables and fruits (including citrus fruits) are the most alkaline.

■ Fasting, prolonged bed rest, lack of exercise, large doses of Vitamin C and synthetic drugs also can create abnormal acid-

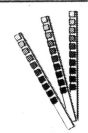

ity and alter pH. Antacids usually produce abnormally alkaline urine, so be sure to take these factors into account when doing pH testing.

■ Be sure that the container you use for collecting your urine sample for pH testing is DRY and clean (this is true for all dipstick tests). Any liquid in the collecting cup other than the urine will change the pH and give you a false test result.

■ Use only freshly voided urine for testing.

INTERPRETING YOUR TEST RESULTS

YOU MUST PERFORM THE PH TEST FOR SEVERAL CONSECUTIVE DAYS IN ORDER TO DETERMINE ABNORMAL pH PATTERNS. Because everyone's pH changes so often during the day, it's crucial to test yourself frequently over the course of several days in order to determine your particular pH pattern.

NORMAL: The normal pattern is a pH that ranges from about 4.5 - 5.5 (morning urine) to 5.5 - 7.0 (afternoon urine) to 7.0 - 8.0 (evening urine). These are not exact pH measurements, but your urine should show fluctuations somewhere in these ranges each day, if you are eating or resting normally.

ABNORMAL: **ACID URINE pH:** After testing your urine pH for 3 - 4 times a day over the course of 7-10 days if you find that your pH is continually very acid (5.5 - 6.0 or below throughout the day) AND you have eliminated obvious factors that can normally affect the test (see previous page), your acid pH tests may indicate:

■ Kidney disorder

51

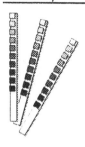

SYMPTOMS OF ACIDOSIS

Symptoms of chronic acidosis include:

- insomnia
- water retention
- frequent sighing
- recessed eyes
- migraine headaches
- abnormally low blood pressure
- rheumatoid arthritis
- dry, hard, foul-smelling stools
- alternating diarrhea and constipation
- sensitivity of the teeth to acid fruits or vinegar

- Diabetes
- Heart or circulatory disease
- Lung disorders that interfere with transfer of oxygen from the lungs to the bloodstream.
- Infection at some location in the body
- *Chronic acidosis:* This condition is caused by habitual improper over-eating of acid foods such as meat and sweets, lack of exercise or excessive stress, obesity, dieting, anger, excess niacin, vitamin C and aspirin.

ALKALINE URINE: If your urine pH test shows a continual pattern of alkalinity (readings of 6.5 and above throughout the day for several days), your tests may indicate:

- Excessive intake of alkaline drugs such as sodium bicarbonate or other similar treatments for ulcers, acid stomach or gastritis.
- High cholesterol
- Endocrine Imbalance
- Poor diet
- Osteoarthritis
- Excessive vomiting (bulimia) and diarrhea can cause alkaline urine
- Stomach or intestinal problems (such as insufficient hydrochloric acid).
- *Chronic Alkalosis:* This is a condition that can result from any of the problems listed above.

IF YOUR TEST IS POSITIVE

 If your pH tests appear continually to be abnormal, check all other test pads for positive results (particularly GLUCOSE and PROTEIN).

2 If no other positive tests are noted on the Multistix dip-stick, continue testing your pH several times each day for 10 days to 2 weeks. For frequent daily pH testing, it's cheaper and more precise to use separate pH papers (see order form in back). Record each pH reading and then review after 10 days to 2 weeks to see if abnormal pH patterns are occurring.

3 If you observe a pattern of abnormal pH, make dietary adjustments and then check your pH readings again.

4 If you have a continually **acid** test result (below 6.0), eat more fresh vegetables, grains and fruits. Avoid meat, fish, poultry, eggs, over-cooked and fried foods, coffee, tea (herbal is fine) and sugar.

If you have a continually **alkaline** test result (6.5 and above), eat more beans, grains, fish and cooked vegetables. Avoid excess raw foods, sugars, and fruits.

5 If you observe a continual pattern of abnormal pH readings that do not improve after dietary adjustments, report the test results to your health practitioner. Make sure you have a written record of your pH readings which have been taken over the course of 10 days to 2 weeks.

SYMPTOMS OF ALKALOSIS

Symptoms of chronic alkalosis include:

- sore muscles
- creaking joints
- bursitis
- bone or heel spurs
- drowsiness
- protruding eyes
- hypertension
- seizures
- edema
- allergies
- night cramps
- asthma
- chronic hyperventilation
- menstrual problems
- night coughs
- chronic indigestion or vomiting
- dry, hard stools
- inflammation of the prostate
- itching skin
- overexcitability of the nervous system

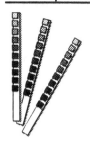

VI. BLOOD

The test on the Multistix 10 for blood is done primarily to detect blood in the urine which is not visible. Visible blood does occasionally appear in the urine in cases of bladder infections, cystitis, excessive exercise (marathons) or menstruation, but the Multistix dipstick test is for detecting invisible blood that may indicate disorders such as kidney stones, infections or other disease conditions.

The condition of having hidden (or occult blood) in the urine can be an extremely important indicator of a health problem and any positive dipstick test needs to be reported to your health practitioner.

BEST TIME FOR TESTING

Your urine can be tested for occult (hidden) blood at any time during the day.

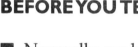

BEFORE YOU TEST CONSIDER THIS:

■ Normally, no blood should appear in the urine and your urine dipstick test for blood should appear negative. A positive test may occur during menstruation, so a second test should be done a few days after menstruation to confirm that the positive test for blood was caused by menstrual blood in the urine and is not due to an underlying disorder.

■ Large amounts of Vitamin C may affect the outcome of your test, so stop your Vitamin supplements 1-2 days before testing (this is a good idea for urine dipstick testing in general).

■ Many individuals will regularly test positive for blood in the urine because of an inherited condition sometimes referred to as familial hematuria. Check with your health practitioner before you decide that this is the reason for a positive test result for blood in the urine.

INTERPRETING YOUR TEST RESULTS:

NORMAL: The test pad for BLOOD on your dipstick should appear as gold (or Negative) after being dipped in the urine (see the first color block on the color chart in the Blood column). Be sure you have waited 60 seconds before reading your results.

ABNORMAL: If the BLOOD pad on your dipstick is any color other than gold (Negative), your urine does contain some invisible (occult) blood.

Non-Hemolyzed:
The color blocks that have the words "Non-Hemolyzed" above them indicate that the blood cells in your urine are whole, intact red blood cells. The condition of having whole red blood cells in your urine is known as "hematuria".

Hemolyzed:
The word "Hemolyzed" means that the red blood cells in your urine have been ruptured, or broken down. Normally, old red blood cells die off or rupture and release hemoglobin (a protein compound in the blood that carries oxygen to the cells). This process is called "hemolysis". However, these ruptured red blood cells (or their hemoglobin) do not normally appear in the urine.

When the urine dipstick test is positive for Hemolyzed Blood (Trace, small, moderate or large), it usually indicates that there is an infec-

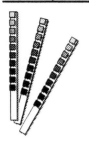

tion, or other problem in your kidneys or urinary tract that has caused ruptured red blood cells (or hemoglobin) to appear in your urine. Some urine dipsticks have the word 'hemoglobin' above certain color blocks which means the same thing as 'hydrolyzed'. The condition of having hemoglobin (or 'hemolyzed' blood cells) in your urine is known as "hemoglobinuria".

IF YOUR TEST IS POSITIVE

1 A positive urine dipstick test for BLOOD may indicate bleeding in the urinary tract possibly caused by:

- Kidney stones
- Kidney inflammation or infection
- Urinary tract infection or inflammation (in the ureters, urethra or bladder)
- Prostate infection
- Malignancy or tumor somewhere in the kidney, urinary tract or prostate
- Liver disorder
- Auto-immune disorders such as lupus
- Anemia

2 Report any positive test results for Blood in the urine to your health practitioner immediately.

3 If your Blood test is positive, check these other dipstick test pads for positive results:

- Check the Protein, the Leukocyte, and the Nitrite test pads (which could help indicate or confirm the blood in the urine is caused by an infection in the kidney or elsewhere in the urinary tract) .

■. Check Urobilinogen and Bilirubin test pads (which could indicate a problem in the liver or elsewhere that is causing an abnormal destruction of red blood cells).

■ Be certain to make a note of any positive test readings on the dipstick that accompany the positive Blood test and report all test results to your health practitioner.

■. After beginning any treatment that might follow your positive test, continue to monitor yourself with the urine dipstick so that you can track your progress.

VII. SPECIFIC GRAVITY

Specific Gravity is a test of how well your kidneys function and can reveal a wealth of crucial health information.

Throughout each day, your kidneys sort through all the nutrients, substances and fluids in your blood. The kidneys remove excess water and nutrients when not immediately needed through your urine. Fluids and nutrients that are needed are returned to the blood by the kidneys. This kidney function balances every element properly in your blood and allows you to function.

Because your kidneys are so critical to maintaining life and health, it's important to monitor how well they're working. One way we can do this is by observing and measuring the Specific Gravity of our urine. This is how Specific Gravity works:

Your first morning urine usually looks very yellow and concentrated. This is because the kidneys have conserved your body fluids during the night when you ordinarily are not taking in fluids, so less fluid has been deposited in the urine. This concentrated morning urine contains less fluid, so the solids are

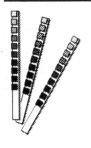

more concentrated, which gives morning urine its characteristic dark yellow appearance. Urine that is low in fluids, but high in solids has a HIGH SPECIFIC GRAVITY.

As you eat and drink through the day, you take in fluids, and the kidneys deposit excess fluid in the urine. Now your urine contains more fluid and the solids are more diluted, which gives the urine a lighter yellow color (LOW SPECIFIC GRAVITY).

When testing for Specific Gravity, you're looking for PATTERNS of abnormalities. An occasional test which seems to be abnormal is not a good indication of a problem. Frequent dipstick testing that shows abnormal Specific Gravity should be reported to your health practitioner for further evaluation.

BEST TIME FOR TESTING

The Specific Gravity test can be performed at any time during the day (see below for more instructions).

BEFORE YOU TEST CONSIDER THIS:

■ Remember that fluid intake directly affects the Specific Gravity Test. Drinking fluids during the night will give you a lower than normal specific gravity reading in the morning, because your morning urine will be more diluted.

■ Exercise, vomiting, diarrhea and fasting will produce a higher than normal specific gravity reading during the day because your kidneys will be conserving needed water, and so your urine will contain less fluid and more concentrated solids.

■ Because your Specific Gravity changes during the day, test yourself 2-3 times (morning, afternoon and evening) for at least 2 days so that you can observe the normality of abnormality of the pattern of your specific gravity.

INTERPRETING YOUR TEST RESULTS:

The color blocks in the Specific Gravity column on the color chart range from dark green to orange and there is a number above each block.

NORMAL: Morning urine should turn the Specific Gravity test pad a greenish-orange to orange color (approximately 1.025 to 1.030). This is a high specific gravity because your morning urine is normally more concentrated (no fluid intake during sleep).

Afternoon and evening urine should produce a light green to greenish orange color on the specific gravity test pad (approximately 1.010 - 1.020).

The most important thing to look for in **testing** Specific Gravity is change. The specific **gravity** of your urine should always change in **response** to fluid intake AND SHOULD RANGE FROM APPROXIMATELY 1.025 (morning.) to 1.010 (afternoon or evening with normal eating and drinking):

■ less fluid intake = higher Specific Gravity (1.020 - 1.025 range)

■ more fluids intake = lower Specific Gravity (1.010 - 1.015 range).
(The numerical ranges given above are only approximate and will differ slightly for every individual).

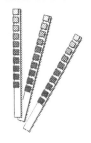

ABNORMAL: Abnormal Specific Gravity readings are:

■ CONTINUAL LOW SPECIFIC GRAVITY THROUGHOUT THE DAY:

Repeated test results which show only continual low specific gravity (approximately 1.000 to 1.005 from morning until night every day even with normal eating and drinking) can indicate:

■ Diabetes insipidus:
a disease caused by a hormone imbalance in which large amounts of watery urine are excreted continually throughout the day.

■ Kidney disease or damage including:
Inflammation or infection in the kidney referred to as nephritis, glomerulonephritis or pyelonephritis.

■ Structural damage to the renal (kidney) tubes.

II. CONTINUAL HIGH SPECIFIC GRAVITY THROUGHOUT THE DAY:

Repeated test results over several days which show only high specific gravity readings (approximately 1.020 to 1.030 from morning until night with normal eating and drinking) can indicate:

■ Adrenal insufficiency
■ Liver Disease
■ Congestive Heart Failure
■ Excessive sweating, fever, vomiting or diarrhea

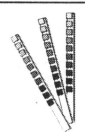

IF YOUR TEST IS POSITIVE

1 Again, it's important to test for Specific Gravity for several days (at least 3-4 days) in order to get accurate test results. Record each of your test results and show the record to your doctor if a pattern of abnormal Specific Gravity readings appear.

2 Check all other test pads for positive results, particularly the GLUCOSE and PROTEIN test pads. These tests may confirm that the abnormal specific gravity is due to possible diabetes (Glucose) or kidney dysfunction (Protein). Report any positive test results along with your record of Specific Gravity readings to your health practitioner for further evaluation.

VIII. KETONES

Fat metabolism is very much connected to carbohydrate metabolism. If you are not eating enough carbohydrates, or if your system isn't using carbohydrates properly, your body soon begins to use increasing amounts of available fatty acids. This places a strain on the system, and now fat metabolism becomes impaired.

When this happens, acids called KETONES appear in the blood and are excreted in the urine. These ketones (or acids) can be detected by the urine dipstick test and tell you and your doctor that something is wrong with your carbohydrate absorption or utilization.

The most common disorder in carbohydrate metabolism is caused by diabetes mellitis.

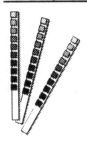

BEST TIME FOR TESTING

The Ketone test can be performed at any time during the day.

BEFORE YOU TEST, CONSIDER THIS:

■ Fasting, dehydration and inadequate food intake can produce a positive test for Ketones, but simply correcting the diet will return the test to normal.

■ Use only fresh, newly collected urine sample for testing.

■ Wait 40 seconds before reading results.

INTERPRETING THE TEST

NORMAL: The first tan color block indicates a Negative test result (no abnormal ketones).

ABNORMAL: A color pad that matches the other color blocks in the Ketone column on the color chart is a positive test for ketones in the urine and may indicate:

■ Too few carbohydrates in the diet from fasting, dieting, poor diet, etc.

■ Early or developing *Diabetes mellitus:* Diabetes mellitus is caused by a lack of insulin secretion by the pancreas, which leads to impaired carbohydrate, fat and protein metabolism. The defect in carbohydrate and fat metabolism produces abnormal ketones in the urine.

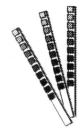

IF YOUR TEST IS POSITIVE

 If your ketone test is positive, make certain that you are eating and drinking normally. Retest yourself after two or three normal meals to see if the Ketone test is now negative.

 Observe the GLUCOSE test pad for any positive results.

 Report all positive test results to your health practitioner.

BILIRUBIN

Bilirubin is formed from the hemoglobin which is normally released by the breakdown of red blood cells after their normal life span (about four months). Once the bilirubin is formed, it combines with protein (albumin) in the bloodstream and is transported to the liver.

In the liver, the bilirubin is broken down and is then excreted into the bowel and solid waste. Bilirubin gives liver bile its gold color and contributes to the black color of solid waste. Unless there is a problem in liver functioning, bilirubin does not normally appear in detectable amounts in the urine.

If there is disease or damage in the liver, bilirubin may not be excreted properly from the body through bile and feces, but instead builds up in improper amounts in the blood. The kidneys will then excrete the bilirubin into the urine, where it can be detected by the urine dipstick test.

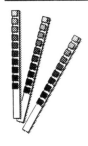

A positive urine test for Bilirubin can detect liver disease and other disorders even before overt symptoms of liver damage appear.

BEST TIME FOR TESTING

The Bilirubin Test can be performed at any time during the day.

BEFORE YOU TEST CONSIDER THIS:

■ Use only a freshly collected urine sample that has not been exposed to bright light for testing.

■ Many different drugs can interfere with the Bilirubin test. Check with your doctor or pharmacist to determine whether a medication you're taking will affect the Bilirubin urine test.

■ Brown urine can indicate abnormal amounts of bilirubin. The yellow color of skin and eyes in jaundice is also caused by excessive amounts of bilirubin and these factors may help you and your doctor to confirm a positive Bilirubin urine test.

INTERPRETING THE TEST

NORMAL: Your Bilirubin test pad on the urine dipstick should show match the first very light beige color block (Negative) after testing.

ABNORMAL: Test results that match the other color blocks in the Bilirubin column may indicate:
■ Gallstones
■ Cirrhosis of the liver or other liver disorder
■ Hepatitis
■ Thyroid disease
■ Cancer

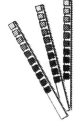

IF YOUR TEST IS POSITIVE:

 Make certain that you are not taking medication that interferes with the test and that you are using a fresh urine sample.

2 Also check the Urobilinogen test pad for positive results.

3 Report all positive Bilirubin test results immediately to your health practitioner.

X. GLUCOSE

The presence of detectable amounts of the sugar, Glucose, in the urine is known as "glycosuria" (gly-cos-ur-ee-ah).. The urine dipstick test for excess sugar in the urine is commonly performed as an early warning signal to detect possible Diabetes mellitus.

In Diabetes mellitus, the body produces decreased levels of the hormone, insulin. Insulin helps in metabolizing carbohydrates and fats, and it also regulates the levels of glucose in the blood. When there is not enough insulin being produced by the pancreas, blood glucose levels rise and this excess glucose is then excreted by the kidneys and ends up in the urine.

We can detect this abnormal glucose in the urine with urine dipstick tests, which can alert us to a possible problem with diabetes. However, an occasional positive Glucose test can indicate something as simple as a heavy meal or excess emotional stress.

 BEST TIME FOR TESTING

Second urination of the morning.

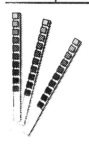
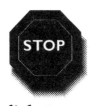

BEFORE YOU TEST, CONSIDER THIS:

Factors that can temporarily produce a positive Glucose test result that does not necessarily indicate diabetes:

- Eating large amounts of sugary food before testing.
- Extreme physical exertion
- Emotional stress
- Certain medications (check with your doctor or pharmacist)
- Pregnancy

INTERPRETING THE TEST

NORMAL: The Glucose test pad should match the aqua (Negative) color block on the color chart.

ABNORMAL: All other color blocks on the color chart indicate abnormal detectable amounts of glucose in the urine. The darker the color block is (from green to brown), the more glucose there is in the urine.

IF THE TEST IS POSITIVE

1 Make certain that you have eliminated all non-disease factors that can influence the Glucose test (listed in Before You Test).

2 Retest yourself 2-3 times each day for 4-5 days and record each test result.

3 If you see a pattern of abnormal Glucose test results appear, report the results to your health practitioner and show your written record to the physician for further evaluation.

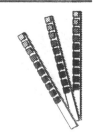

Now that you've learned how to interpret each test on the Multistix 10 dipsticks, we're going to go over the step-by-step process of performing the urine dipstick test.

DIRECTIONS FOR USING THE AMES (MILES) MULTISTIX 10 URINE DIPSTICKS

1 Collect the urine sample by means of a clean catch (see pages 37 and 38).

2 Use only freshly voided (passed) urine for testing.

3 The best time for general testing is on first urination in the morning, although certain tests should be repeated at different times during the day to best determine results. This includes Specific Gravity, pH, Glucose, Ketones and Protein tests (see information under individual tests in this chapter for more information on testing times).

4 Dip the test strip into the urine sample for no more than 1 second. Make sure that you have immersed the entire strip in the urine.

5 Draw the edge of the strip along the rim of the specimen container to remove any excess urine.

6 Turn the test strip on its side and tap once on a piece of absorbent paper (tissue) to remove any remaining urine and to prevent the possible mixing of reagent chemicals from pad to pad. Then lay the dipstick (pads up) on a clean tissue.

7 Using a clock with a second hand, begin reading the test results at the appropriate time (see below). To read test results, hold the dipstick by long plastic end that contains

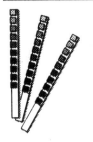

no pads and simply compare the colors of the dipstick pads to the color chart. Your fingers holding the dipstick should be at the bottom of the color chart (Glucose) so that the pads are correctly aligned with the color chart.

1. 30 seconds after dipping, observe:
   - ■ Bilirubin pad
   - ■ Glucose pad

2. 40 seconds after dipping observe:
   - ■ Ketone pad

3. 45 seconds after dipping observe:
   - ■ Specific Gravity pad

4. 60 seconds (1 minute) after dipping observe these pads:
   - ■ Blood
   - ■ pH
   - ■ Protein
   - ■ Urobilinogen
   - ■ Nitrite

5. 2 minutes (120 seconds) after dipping observe:
   - ■ Leukocyte pad

The timing of reading the test results after dipping do not have to be absolutely exact, but try to get it as close as possible. In order to do this, it's best to be prepared ahead of time by reading over this entire chapter on dipsitck testing BEFORE you test, so that you can know what you're doing and what the test results mean as you're comparing the dipstick to the color chart after dipping.

Once you've become familiar with how to use and interpret the urine dipstick screening tests, you'll have powerful tool right at

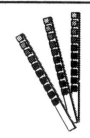

your fingertips for monitoring your own health right at home with the same professional accuracy that doctors use for their screening tests.

Now that you've learned a modern way of testing for health problems at home, we're going to look in the next chapter at a very ancient, but highly effective method of monitoring abnormalities in the body that can help indicate or alert you to present or potential illnesses or disease.

CHAPTER FOUR:
MORE DIAGNOSTIC TESTS

THE URINE CALCIUM TEST

IN THIS CHAPTER

■ The Urine Calcium Test

■ Blood Pressure

■ The Lung Check Test

Calcium is an extremely important mineral that maintains several critical functions in our bodies. Calcium maintains cell structure, blood clotting, nerve functions, muscle contraction and prevents vitamin D toxicity or deficiency.

Too little or too much calcium in the body can cause many different types of disorders. Inadequate levels of calcium can lead to disorders such as bone thinning and deterioration (osteoporosis), while excessive calcium can contribute to kidney stones and other health problems.

Urine testing for calcium in the body is simple and is an excellent indicator of how much calcium you're getting in your diet AND how much of your dietary calcium you are assimilating. Measuring urine calcium can also reflect hormonal disorders such as thyroid and parathyroid imbalances which directly affect the level of calcium in the body.

The most common test for urine calcium is called the Sulkowitch test (named for the American doctor who invented the test). This test is not a dipstick test but is performed by adding the Sulkowitch powder or liquid reagent to your urine sample and observing its effect on the clarity of the urine (how cloudy it becomes after reagent is added).

BEFORE YOU TEST CONSIDER THIS:

■ Certain drugs or medications can affect calcium levels. Antacids, diuretics, large doses of vitamin D, laxatives, some antibiotics and birth control pills can alter calcium levels in the body. So if you're taking a medication, check with your pharmacist or health practitioner before taking the Sulkowitch urine calcium test.

■ Avoid Soft drinks, or sodas for at least 24-36 hours before testing. Sodas contain excessive phosphates which decrease body calcium and will affect the results of the Sulkowitch calcium test.

■ Check your urine for protein before testing for calcium, especially if you suspect you have a kidney problem. Protein in the urine can make the urine cloudy, so it will be difficult to tell whether it's the protein or the calcium test that is causing the urine cloudiness.

■ If you have a urinary tract infection, it can turn the urine cloudy and interfere with the results of the calcium test. Take the calcium test once your infection has been healed.

■ The Sulkowitch powder or liquid reagent is a mixture of two potent acids. KEEP POWDER OUT OF REACH OF CHILDREN, DO NOT ingest the reagent and DO NOT let the powder or liquid reagent come into contact with your skin, clothes or furniture.

TAKING THE TEST

Collect the urine specimen approximately one hour after a typical meal. (This can be breakfast, lunch or dinner). It is not necessary to do a clean or midstream catch.

Pour 1/4 cup of urine into a clean, clear glass that you do not intend to use for anything other than the calcium test. The reagent should never be ingested, so it's best to simply set aside a special small glass that you use only for the Sulkowitch calcium test.

FOR LIQUID: Add 2 drops of liquid to 1/4 cup urine

FOR POWDER: Add 1 teaspoon powder to 1 teaspoon urine

INTERPRETING THE TEST

When you add the Sulkowitch reagent (powder or liquid) to the urine, the urine should show some degree of cloudiness. The degree of cloudiness indicates the amount of calcium in the urine:

■ No cloudiness is given a rating of 0 and indicates that no measurable amount of calcium is in the urine.

■ Slightly cloudy to a heavier cloudiness (you can still read the printing on a label, newspaper or book through the glass containing the urine) is given a rating of 1+ to 2+ and indicates a normal amount of calcium in the urine.

■ Very cloudy (cannot read or see through the glass containing the urine sample) is given a rating of 3+ to 4+ and indicates excessive calcium in the urine.

This is how to interpret how much calcium is in the urine sample:

NORMAL: Slightly cloudy (printed matter still visible through the specimen glass — 1+ to 2+) indicates normal/adequate intake and utilization of calcium.

ABNORMAL: **No Cloudiness (0):** Insufficient Calcium in the diet or poor assimilation and utilization of ingested calcium.

Abnormally low levels of calcium in the urine may indicate:

- Lack of sufficient calcium in the diet

- Intestinal problems (poor digestion or assimilation)

- hormone imbalance

- kidney disease

- nutritional deficiencies

- Excessive ingestion of soft drinks (soda)

WHAT TO DO:
If your first calcium test produces no cloudiness, eat another meal containing no calcium and retest. Later eat another meal containing large amounts of calcium-rich foods and supplements and then retest again. Retest again later after ingesting another calcium-rich meal.

If each test produces an uncloudy urine sample, it could be an early warning sign of osteoporosis or other health problem. Write down a record of your test results, along with what foods you ate before each test and report the results to your doctor for further evaluation.

Extremely Cloudy *(Cannot see or read through the specimen glass) (3+ - 4+)*: Excessive Calcium in the diet or abnormal calcium excretion

Excessive calcium in the urine may indicate:

■ You've eaten a calcium rich meal or ingested calcium supplements within a few hours of taking the test, in which case, it is normal for the calcium test to turn the urine very cloudy.

■ Kidney stones or kidney problems

■ Hormonal or other problem which is causing abnormal excretion of calcium.

WHAT TO DO:
If your first test produces very cloudy urine, retest yourself after eating one or two meals that do not contain calcium- rich foods and do not take supplements at least 24 hours before the test. If this second test still produces very cloudy urine, retest once again following the same instructions (eliminating calcium).

If the third test produces very cloudy urine, report your test results to your health practitioner (make sure that you report what time of day you took the test and what diet you ingested before each test).

ACCURACY

The Sulkowitch test for urine calcium is about 80% accurate in detecting an underlying disease or health problem that is interfering with calcium utilization in the body, and is the same test that doctors and laboratories perform for calcium level screening, particularly for osteoporosis.

BLOOD PRESSURE

Monitoring your blood pressure is one of the most important home tests you can do, especially as you get older. With today's new digital monitors, it's easier than ever to keep track of your blood pressure and to monitor or avert possible heart and cardiovascular diseases.

USING A BLOOD PRESSURE MONITOR

1. The best blood pressure monitors for home use are the monitors that come with a digital display and don't require the use of a stethoscope. These digital monitors automatically display your blood pressure reading which makes for much easier, more accurate readings.

2. Follow the directions that come with the monitor carefully. It's best to place the blood pressure cuff on your bare upper arm. Make sure that your arm is not constricted by clothing, and don't place clothing over the monitor.

3. Take your blood pressure while sitting down. Rest your forearm on a table, with the cuff at heart level.

Pump the air pump with your free hand, NOT with the hand of the arm that is wrapped with the cuff.

 If the cuff does not automatically deflate (most of the new ones do), make sure to let the air out of the cuff slowly and evenly.

UNDERSTANDING BLOOD PRESSURE MEASUREMENTS

When the doctor tells you your blood pressure is, for instance, 140 over 90, it means that blood pressure at the moment the heart contracts is 140. The pressure at the moment the heart is resting is 90. These functions are referred to as systolic and diastolic blood pressure:

Systolic Pressure:	Heart contracts (forcing blood from heart into the arteries). High point of blood pressure.
Diastolic Pressure:	Momentary resting phase of the heart. High point of blood pressure.
Example:	(Blood pressure 140 over 90) 140/90 Systolic pressure / Diastolic pressure

In taking your blood pressure, you need to repeat the test several times in order to see a pattern. The exception to this is if ANY blood pressure reading is over 180.

Take your blood pressure for at least 3 times a day for three days.

INTERPRETING THE TEST

NORMAL: Blood pressure normally fluctuates throughout the day, depending on your level of activity. Blood pressure normally goes up with physical exertion, and decreases during times of rest and relaxation.

In general, normal blood pressure is 120/80 (120 over 80).

ABNORMAL: **High Blood Pressure (Hypertension):** Repeated, consistent systolic readings higher than 150 and/or diastolic readings higher than 90. Report repeated blood pressure reading over 150/90 to your doctor immediately.

Abnormally high blood pressure can indicate:

- Heart disease

- Blockage or obstruction in arteries

- Kidney disease

- Connective tissue disease

- Nervous system disorder

- Lung disorders or disease

- Hormonal problems

Low Blood Pressure (Hypotension): Repeated consistent systolic readings below 100 and diastolic readings below 65 should be reported to your doctor.

Abnormally Low Blood Pressure Can Indicate:

■ Side effect of drugs and medications (diuretics and tranquilizers)

■ Parkinson's-type diseases

■ Nervous system disorders

■ Internal bleeding

ACCURACY

Studies have actually shown that blood pressure tests done at home, when done properly, are more accurate (95%) than those performed in a doctor's office. Stress, anxiety or overexcitement during doctor's visits often result in erroneous blood pressure readings.

In recent years, average blood pressures have reportedly dropped as much as 10% since people began testing their own blood pressure at home.

THE LUNG CHECK TEST

Lung cancer and lung problems due to smoking, air pollutants, pesticides and chemical sprays have become a real health hazard in our modern day world. Lung cancer and respiratory problems are widespread, and we need to be conscientious about monitoring the health condition of our lungs. Early diagnosis of lung irritation or changes in lung tissues and cells can make a huge difference in catching and arresting lung disorders before they develop into big health problems.

One of the best tests that I've come across for monitoring the condition of the lungs is called the Lung Check Test. This is one of the simplest and most powerful ways to check your lungs that I've ever seen and can be done simply by ordering the test and providing a sputum (or saliva) sample.

The thing that most impressed me about this test is that it can detect extremely subtle, minute changes in lung cells or tissue that are an early warning of lung cancer, lung disease, irritation, etc.

Reportedly, this test is one of the most powerful early detection systems around for lung problems, and is said to be far more effective than x-rays or other diagnostic tests for lung disease, because it detects lung problems at the cellular level, before they're serious or advanced enough to be detected through x-rays or doctor's exams. Also, the test is FDA approved.

HOW TO TAKE THE TEST

From what I've been told, you can order the test yourself, which saves you the inflated pricing and time at the doctor's office. A container for the sputum sample and the directions for taking the test are mailed to you, and then you simply provide the sample and mail the labeled container back to the address provided.

In 7-10 days, a report (see below) is mailed back to you which details all of your test results. There are several graphs and interpretations, most of which are self-explanatory. You can then take the test results to your health practitioner if the test results indicate a problem or for a more in-depth explanations of the results.

INTERPRETING THE TEST

The Lung Check Test results will indicate:

- Any lung irritation from smoking, allergies, chemicals, etc.

- Asthma (early or developed)

- Bronchitis (early or advanced)

- Lung cancer (even at the earliest stages before tumors develop)

- Changes in the cells and tissues of the lungs due to any form of lung disease.

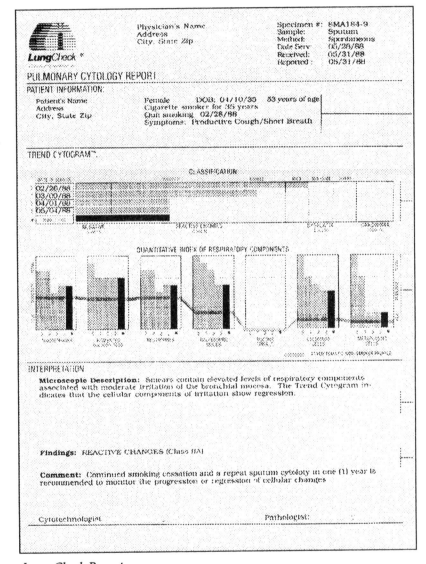

Lung Check Report

Your Lung test is evaluated by qualified, certified pathologists and cytotechnologists (technicians who evaluate cellular changes in the body). If any part of your test results indicates abnormalities, take the written test results to your doctor for further evaluation.

ORDERING THE TEST

You can get more information on ordering the Lung Check Test by calling FutureMed, Inc. in Arizona at 1-800-800-8849, or write to them at:

FutureMed, Inc.
Box 13837
Scottsdale, AZ   85267

CHAPTER FIVE:
YOUR BODY'S TALKING

I n Western medicine, we've come to rely so heavily on high-tech diagnostic machines and complicated "objective' medical tests, that we completely overlook the sometimes very obvious signals of illness and disease that are right in front of our nose—literally.

For thousands of years, Eastern medicine has incorporated minute observations of the appearance of the body itself in diagnosing disease. And it makes sense. Any illness or abnormality in the body is going to produce changes in tissues, organs, cells, etc., and it's obvious that sooner or later these internal changes in the body are going to show up externally.

Most of us are aware that extremely obvious external abnormalities like tumors, rashes, ulcers and so on signal disease or illness in the body. But what about more subtle signs that might help us to diagnose and prevent a disease before it becomes a real problem?

Well, fortunately, there is a whole body of knowledge given to us from the East that teaches us how to interpret the language of the body——the signs and early warning signals of illness that can be diagnosed painlessly, simply by knowing what your body appearance is telling you about the state of your health.

**IN THIS
CHAPTER**

■ General
Appearance/
Constitution

■ Specific
Characteristics

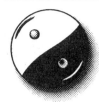

Now, the amount of information on diagnosing the body appearance is huge, and I'm not going to try to duplicate what's taken thousands of years to compile. But in this chapter, we're going to review a few of the most useful external-body diagnostic techniques that will give you a step up on learning more about what your body can tell you about your health.

THE FIRST STEP

One of the first steps in understanding Eastern medicine, (on which all of the information in this chapter is based), is to try to grasp the meaning of the words Yin and Yang.

As Oriental medicine has become more integrated into Western culture through acupuncture, acupressure, Chinese herbs, etc., we Westerners have generally become more familiar with these terms, but frankly, they're complicated. Because the terms Yin and Yang encompass a number of different meanings which embody a whole philosophy of Eastern medicine, simplifying the understanding of what it all means to the Western mind can be difficult.

I've chosen just a few of the underlying meanings of Yin and Yang so that you can get a flavor of how these principles are applied to diagnosing your body's appearance. My explanations of Yin and Yang are very abbreviated here so that you'll have a simplified approach to the techniques of Oriental diagnosis. If you find that you want to study the principles of Yin and Yang and Oriental medicine more deeply, there are many excellent in-depth guides that can help you. I particularly recommend Paul Pitchford's book, Healing With Whole Foods. This 650 page how- to guide leaves nothing unsaid about how to use Eastern medicine in the Western world.

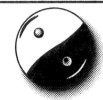

So start studying your body language (and your family's)! You'll find it pays to be attentive to the health tips your appearance can reveal.

	Physical Characteristics	Mental/Emotional Characteristics
Yin:	More delicate constitution	Sensitive, artistic, more introverted, inclined to be more mentally active
Yang	Stronger, more robust constitution	Outgoing, aggressive, extroverted, more physically and socially active

Good, normal health = balanced amounts of yin and yang tendencies

Health abnormalities = excessive yin or yang caused by:

- Inherited characteristics

- Dietary imbalances:

- Excessive meats, grains, salts = Too Yang

- Excessive fruits, vegetable, sweets = Too Yin

GENERAL APPEARANCE / CONSTITUTION

FAMILY INFLUENCES ON HEALTH

Knowing which parental characteristics we may have inherited can give us keys to our own health tendencies. By observing our parent's health and applying the following guides, we can make changes in our own health regimens that can help us

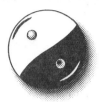

overcome inherited weaknesses and possibly prevent them from manifesting as diseases later in life:

Father influences: Child's nervous system
Intellectual, ideological character
Social interactions and characteristics
Left side of the body:
    Left lung, left heart atrium, spleen, pancreas, stomach
    Left kidney, left side of small intestine, descending colon, left ovary or testicle

Mother influences: Child's digestive and reproductive system
Physical character
Emotional characteristics
Right side of the body:
    Right lung, right heart atrium, liver, gallbladder, right kidney, duodenum
    Right side of small intestine, ascending colon, right ovary or testicle

BODY SIZE

Thin & Tall = Yin Tendencies

Thin & Short = More sensitive health

More mental and withdrawn

More susceptible to respiratory and nervous disorders

Tall & Robust = Yang tendencies

Short & Stocky = Stronger health
Active physical & social lives

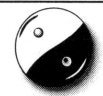

More susceptible to digestive
and circulatory disorders

HEAD SIZE

Large head = Stronger than average constitution
More aggressive behavior
Socially outgoing

Small head = More delicate, weaker constitution
Tends to be more introverted,
    sensitive and artistic
Tendency towards weaker health

SHOULDERS

Square shoulders = More masculine characteristics
Physically and socially active
    and outgoing

Round, sloping = More feminine characteristics
shoulders   Sensitive, artistic nature

One shoulder = Weakened organs on the side
higher than   of higher shoulder
another   Weakness in lungs and large intestines

BONES

Strong, large bones = Strong constitution
Active physical and social life

Small, thin bones = Weaker, more fragile health
(constitution)
More mental and artistic tendencies

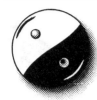

WALK

Normal walk = Feet parallel when walking

Abnormal = Toes point in (pigeon-toed): Too Yang
Excessive meat, salt

Toes point out: Too Yin
Excessive fruits & sugars

Bowlegged: Too Yang
Excessive meat & salt

POSTURE

Erect posture = Stronger health
More robust (Yang) constitution

Slumping posture = Weaker, more sensitive health

SPECIFIC CHARACTERISTICS

MOUTH

Good Health = Mouth which is same width
or narrower than the width of the nose.

Large mouth = Overall weaker organs and glands
The modern diet (too many sweets,
weaker immune responses meats,
coffee, oils, & fats) has

Too Yin = increased mouth size in modern man.

Very small mouth = Too Yang (contracted organs)
Excessive meats, grains & salts

LIPS

Good Health = lips of equal, medium thickness

	INDICATE	**POSSIBLE CAUSE**
Thick Lips	stronger than average skin & muscles weaker internal organs (heart, liver, spleen, small intestines).	Excessive grains, refined flours, potatoes, fruits and fats (typical diet in tropical climates)
Thin Lips	weaker endurance and resistance Sensitive, unbalanced constitution	Excessive refined foods, sweets, animal products and processed foods.
Swollen upper lip	enlarged liver stomach disorders	Poor quality of food
Swollen lower lip	Intestinal disorders	
Both lips swollen	Intestinal & stomach disorders	
Yellow crust at corners of lips	digestive problems liver & gallbladder congestion	Excessive saturated fats, meat, poultry, eggs, cheese, etc.

LIP COLOR

Pinkish red = Good health (normal digestion, circulation and lung functions)

Vivid red	=	Blood capillaries expanded, possible respiratory dysfunction, possible elevated blood pressure, or inflammation or infection somewhere in the body.
White	=	Blood capillaries abnormally contracted, deficiency in hemoglobin, anemia, leukemia associated with white lips.
Pinkish white	=	Possible allergies, asthma, skin or hormonal disorders, circulatory or respiratory problems.
		Excessive sugar, fruits, dairy products and fats.
Dark lips	=	kidney & urinary tract dysfunction, liver & gall bladder problems.
		Excessive salts and fatty acids.
Dark red	=	Dysfunction in heart or circulation, lungs, kidney, urinary tract; disorders in liver, gallbladder, spleen and pancreas.
		Excessive salts, proteins and saturated fats.
Dark purple	=	Very poor blood circulation. Advanced organ degeneration (intestines, liver, spleen, kidneys and lungs). May be caused by improper diet.

Black spots   =   Kidney and urinary tract disorders; hardened fats in the digestive tract.

Excessive fruits, sugars and carbohydrates.

White patches   =   Temporary dysfunction of digestive, respiratory and lymphatic system. Excessive dairy products and fats.

TEETH

Buck Teeth   =   Excessive Yin foods during growth years (fruits, sugars, refined foods, raw foods)

Concave (grow inward)   =   Excessive animal products, salts, cooked foodsduring growth years

Crooked Teeth   =   Excessive animal foods, sugar, dairy

Teeth sticking in and out   =   Poor, chaotic diet. Erratic eating patterns during growth.

Spaces between teeth   =   Excessive Yin foods during growth (sugars, fruits, raw and refined foods).

Vertical ridges on tooth surface   =   Lack of or poor assimilation of protein & fat, kidney problems, excessive salt & carbohydrates

Serrated edges on front teeth   =   Kidney problems; lack of protein, digestive problems

Swollen gums   =   Excessive liquids, sugars, fruits, juices and oils

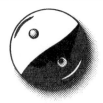

Receding gums = Poor diet. Caused by either Excess animal products & salts or by excess sweets, juices, sodas and processed foods.

Pale, white gums = Poor circulation. Lack of hemoglobin. Possible anemia.

Pimples inside = Improper diet. Too much protein, fat, mouth oils or sugars.

TONGUE

SHAPE

Wide tongue = Sufficient vegetables eaten by mother with round tip during pregnancy. Generally indicates gentle, understanding, harmonious temperament.

Narrow tongue = Excessive animal foods eaten by mother with pointed tip during pregnancy. Generally indicates rigid, tight, aggressive temperament. May be narrow-minded or offensive in manner.

Tongue with cleft = Excessive raw foods (animal and in the middle or tip vegetable) foods eaten by mother during pregnancy. Indicates a tendency to an indecisive, changeable temperament.

TONGUE COLOR

White = Poor circulation, anemia, excessive fats and mucous buildup.

Dark red = Possible ulcer, inflammation or cancer somewhere in the body.

Yellow coating = liver or gallbladder inflammation (excessive bile). Excessive dairy, eggs and poultry.

Purple = Excessive refined foods, sugars, 'junk food' and fruits.

EYEBROWS

Short distance between eyebrows = susceptible to weakness or disorders of the liver, pancreas, kidneys, heart and glands (too much yang food eaten during childhood).

Wide distance between eyebrows = susceptible to weakness or disorders in the lungs, intestines, bladder and gallbladder (excessive fruits, sugars, vegetables, refined foods eaten during childhood)

Eyebrows slant up = susceptible to liver and heart trouble. More yang characteristics (aggressive, perhaps offensive). Habitual overeating of animal foods (meat).

Eyebrows slant down = susceptible to kidney and intestinal problems. Gentle, accepting nature. Low animal food consumption in daily diet during growth.

Smooth, curving eyebrows = good mental and physical balance. Indicates well- balanced diet eaten by mother during pregnancy.

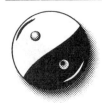

Peaked eyebrows = susceptible to kidney, liver and spleen disorders. Physically and socially active during first years of life. Later in life, more involved with mental and spiritual concerns. Gentle, shy nature. Animal food eaten by mother in first part of pregnancy, more vegetables in second half.

Thick eyebrows = Yang character. Robust, strong health and constitution. Vigorous, active, outgoing personality.

Thin eyebrows = Yin character. Sensitive, artistic, weaker constitution and health.

Very thin eyebrows = Extreme yin character (physically and mentally sensitive and delicate). Proneness to cancer.

Long hair in eyebrows = mentally and spiritually inclined.

Short hair in eyebrows = Inclined to be more physically active.

Broad, full eyebrows = vigorous, active character.

Narrow eyebrows = less physically active; less vitality.

Decreasing eyebrow width = physical and mental degeneration.

Long eyebrows = long life

Short eyebrows = short life

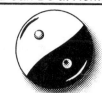

Hair between brows = susceptible to disorders in liver, pancreas and spleen (worsened by excessive animal foods and dairy products.) Caused by excessive intake of meat and dairy by mother during pregnancy.

Spaces in eyebrow hair = May develop serious illness at some point in life.

EYES

Short distance between eyes = Strong, robust physically (Yang). Susceptible to problems in liver, pancreas, spleen and kidney, especially when excess animal foods are eaten. May be aggressive, stubborn and narrow-minded. Intellectually keen. More animal foods and grain eaten during mother's pregnancy.

Wide distance between eyes = Sensitive, more delicate physical and emotional nature (yin). Susceptible to problems in the kidneys, intestines and stomach, especially if excess fruits, sugars, raw or refined foods are eaten. Indicates a gentle character, more mental, less physically active. Tendency to be indecisive.

Eyes slant upwards = Indicate clear, well-balanced emotional and intellectual character. Good balance of grains and salts eaten by mother during pregnancy.

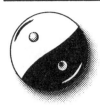

Eyes slant down=Gentle, accepting nature. More fruits, vegetables and raw foods eaten during mother's pregnancy.

Small Eyes = Determined, self-confident, vigorous character. Good physical strength and endurance. Indicates yang diet of cooked foods (animal and vegetables) during mother's pregnancy and formative years.

Very small eyes = Excessively yang temperament. Aggressive, often offensive character.

Large eyes = Delicate, sensitive, gentle nature. Mentally active. Indicates yin diet of fruits, juices, raw foods and sugars eaten during mother's pregnancy and formative years.

Very large eyes = Sensitive nervous system. Tendency to be nervous, irritable, timid and extremely sensitive.

EYELASHES

Long eyelashes = Sensitive, gentle nature (yin). Indicate excess of fruits, raw foods, sugars, vegetables in mother's diet and during formative years.

Short eyelashes = More aggressive, outgoing nature. Indicate yang foods (cooked animal and vegetable products, salts, grains, etc) eaten during mother's pregnancy and growth years.

Eyelashes curve out=	Abnormally nervous and sensitive. Problems and degeneration in the reproductive organs. Excessive yin foods, fruits, juices, sweets, refined foods and synthetic drugs taken during childhood.
Eyelashes curve in =	Problems in reproductive organs, especially menstrual cramps or lack of menstruation. Excessive amounts of meat, eggs, salts, poultry and fish, too few grains and vegetables during growth years.
Bags under the eyes=	1. Watery and swollen: Indicate kidney and bladder disorders. Overloaded internal systems resulting in fatigue, forgetfulness, loss of clear judgments and indecision. Excessive intake of liquids, fruits and juices.
	2. Fatty and swollen: Indicate mucus and fat accumulation in eyebags the kidney tissues signalling the formation of kidney stones. Chronic fat accumulation leading to inflammation in the urinary tact, prostate problems, ovarian cysts and possible tumors or cancers in the reproductive organs.
Dark shadows under the eyes	= Problems with kidneys, lymph system and intestines. Over consumption of salt, liquids and sweets

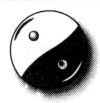

EYEBALL PLACEMENT

Good Health = Eyeball centered in eye with no white showing on top or bottom.

White of eye showing above eyeball = Normal for infants. In adulthood can indicate unbalanced mental functions, or aggressiveness.

White of eye showing below eyeball = Mental and physical health weakened and unbalanced.

NOSE

Shape of the nose indicates brain quality, condition and size.

Normal nose shape = average length and roundness of nose.

Long, straight nose = Sensitive, nervous temperament

Short, flat nose = Determined, sometimes rigid character.

High nose = Tendency to proud, prejudiced, competitive temperament.

Very high, long nose= In women, indicates infertility

Very short flat nose = In men indicates tendency towards violent behavior and poor intelligence.

Enlarged nose = enlarged heart (excessive eating and drinking)

Fat, oily nose = Diet too heavy in animal products

Tip of nose tilts up = Strong, robust, physically and socially active and intellectually keen (yang). May tend to be narrow- minded or shortsighted. Excessive diet of animal foods.

Pointed nose = Nervous temperament, weak heart (yin). Excessive diet of fruits.

Swollen nose = Disorders in circulation and kidneys. Excessive intake of sugars, liquids, fruits,

fats and oils.

Cleft at tip of nose = Irregular heartbeat or heart murmur. Excessive diet of sugars, fruits, juices and soda.

Large nostrils = strong lungs. Determined, strong, more masculine character.

Very large nostrils = Tendency towards violence.

Small nostrils = Gentle, sensitive, more feminine qualities

Very small nostrils = weak lungs

Red blood vessels = high blood pressure, leading to
on tip of nose   heart disease

Purple nose = low blood pressure; possibility of future heart failure.

White nose color = Contraction of the hear and blood vessels, cold fingers, toes and skin.

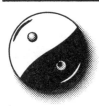

CHEEKS

Represent the condition of the respiratory and circulatory functions.

Good health	=	Well developed, firm cheeks with clean, clear skin.
Thin cheek flesh	=	Weakened respiratory and digestive functions.
Red or pink cheeks	=	Abnormal expansion of capillaries (heart or circulation problems). Excessive yin foods (sugars, fruits, refined foods, alcohol, etc.
Dark spots on cheeks	=	fat or mucous accumulating in lungs (possible the early warning of cyst or tumor formation
Freckles on cheeks	=	Problems with the lungs and digestion. Excessive sugars in the diet (refined sugar, fruits sugar, etc.)

EARS

Ears	=	overall physical and metal constitution, especially kidneys.
Normal	=	Top of ears are level with the eyes, earlobes end at the mouth
Large ears	=	Robust, strong constitution
small ears	=	weaker mental and physical constitution. Excessive animal foods

and flour products during mother's pregnancy.

Small earlobes = weakened nervous system functions. Diet lacking in minerals.

Pointed ears = Excess animal protein. Tendency towards aggressive, sometimes narrow-minded attitudes.

Ears close = good physical and mental health. Good, to the head   well balanced diet eaten by mother during pregnancy.

Ears separated = More mentally than physically active. from head   More delicate, sensitive constitution. Excessive yin foods (fruits, sugars, raw foods, refined foods, coffee, alcohol, etc.).

FOREHEAD

Normal = clear,

Skin slightly = Problems in the heart, circulatory and swollen   lymph systems. Excessive liquids and fruits.

Oily skin on = Liver, gallbladder and digestive forehead   problems. Excess oils and animal foods in diet.

Horizontal wrinkles= Stress or problems in the digestive, early adulthood   circulatory or nervous system. Excessive liquids, fruits, juices, dairy or oils.

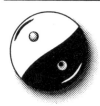

Vertical line between the eyes	=	Accumulation of mucous and fat in the liver. Disorders or dysfunction in liver and gallbladder. Can lead to short tempered, easily upset temperament. Deeper wrinkle indicates more severe condition.

HAIR

Oily hair	=	Excessive fats and oils in diet. May eventually affect respiratory, digestive or reproductive systems.
Dry hair	=	Lack of liquids in diet. Affects liver, gallbladder, spleen, pancreas, circulatory and respiratory functions,
Dandruff	=	Excessive proteins, fats or oils (animal and vegetable). Indicates problems in kidneys and lymph system along with short temper and indecisiveness.
Split ends	=	General overeating of animal foods and sweets. Lack of balanced grains and minerals. Indicates problems in ovaries, uterus, prostate gland and testicles.
Hair loss in front of head	=	Excessive fruits, sweets and liquids (yin foods). Indicates degeneration in heart, circulatory system, kidneys, lymph and reproductive system.
Hair loss from top or back of head	=	Excess animal products (protein), dairy foods and salts (diet too yang). Indicates possible cardiovascular disorders, chronic digestive problems and formation of cysts and tumors.

Hair loss in front = Habitual diet of extreme yang and yin
and back of head   foods (too many animal products,
                     sweets, alcohol, coffee, etc.) Lack of
                     grains, beans and vegetables.Indicates
                     overall degeneration in the body. Often
                     accompanied irritable, changeable
                     temperament.

Grey hair = Liver and gallbladder functions
            becoming underactive. More rigid,
            stubborn personality may develop.

HANDS

PALMS

Palm longer = Strong, robust constitution and health
than fingers

Palm same length = More sensitive, weaker constitution
(or longer) than   and health. More mentally inclined
fingers

Thick, full palm = Strong, (yang) constitution.

Thin, flexible palm = Weaker, more delicate constitution
                      and health

Wide palm = Strong, robust. Potential for long life

Narrow palm = Weaker health. Potential for shorter life

Chronically sweaty = Kidney and lymph system problems,
palms   fatigue, insomnia, forgetfulness and
                     cloudy thinking may be present

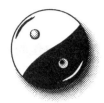

Very dry palms = Too few liquids. Excessive animal foods, grains and salts with too few liquids to balance.

Stiff hands (fingers don't bend back easily) = Congestion or blockage in the arteries (too much cholesterol).

COLOR AT CENTER OF PALM

Red = Circulatory system disorders

Purple = Respiratory and reproductive system disorders

Dark brown   Lymph system and colon disorders

Yellow = Liver and gallbladder disorders

FINGERS

Long, thin fingers = More sensitive, delicate health

Short, thick fingers = Stronger, more robust constitution and health.

Square fingertips = Strong, active, robust, determined and aggressive.

Round fingertips = Active, energetic, positive, understanding, compassionate

Narrow, pointed fingertips = Sensitive, artistic, delicate, spiritually inclined.

Swollen fingertips = Too much overeating of rich animal foods and sweets.

PAIN OR ABNORMALITIES IN OR ON:

Thumb = Problems with lungs

Forefinger = Problems with large intestine

Middle finger = Problems with heart, stomach, circulatory or reproductive functions.

Fourth (ring) finger = Degeneration in body vitality, energy and irregularities in body temperature

Little finger (on palm side) = Problems in heart and circulatory system.

Little finger (backside) = Problems in small intestine and digestive system.

FINGERNAILS

Square nails = Robust, strong, yang constitution. Physically active, may tend to be rigid and inflexible.

Oblong nails = Well-balanced physically and mentally, with tendency towards rigid temperament.

Oval nails = Weaker, more sensitive physical constitution and health. Very active mentally. Emotionally sensitive.

Long nails = Weak physical constitution. Weak lungs and digestive system. Tends to be oversensitive emotionally.

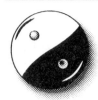

Vertical ridges   =   Excessive carbohydrates and salts.
on nails   Digestive, liver and kidney problems.
                      General fatigue.

White dots   =   Excessive sugars in the diet

Split nails   =   Excessive fruits, sugars, raw foods,
                coffee, alcohol, refined (yin) foods.
                Problems in reproductive system,
                testicles, ovaries, nervous and /
                or circulatory system

Small moons   =   Mentally active, physically weaker.
at base of nail

Larger moons   =   Physically active, less mental personality

Very large moons   =   Physical weakness. Excessive fruits,
                    sugars, juices, coffee, refined foods

THE FEET

Large feet   =   More mental, intellectual and artistic

Small feet   =   Good physical vitality and resistance

FOOT COLOR

Red   =   overactive heart, kidneys and circulatory
        functions. Often accompanied by
        forgetfulness, frequent urination and
        fatigue. Excessive fruits, sweets, refined
        foods and possible medications
        and drugs.

Yellow = Liver and gallbladder disorders.
Excessive animal foods and
vegetable fats

Brown = Underactive kidneys. Excessive animal
foods, flour products and cooked foods.

White = Constricted circulation, heart disorders.
Possible anemia. Excessive animal
products, fats and salts.

TOES

Pain or abnormalities in or on:

Big (first) toe = Liver problems

Second toe = Stomach problems

Third toe = bladder problems

Fourth toe = gallbladder

Fifth (small) toe = the kidneys

TOE SIZE

Second toe = stomach disorders
longer than
big toe

Second and third = Possible stomach disorders, ulcers,
toe longer than   cancer and other diseases.
big toe

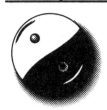

Small, shrunken = Kidney and possible urinary tract
little toe & nail   problems. Constricted, contracted
                     kidneys.

SKIN CONDITION OF FEET

Athlete's foot = Weak or dysfunctional kidneys.
                 Excessive fruits, sugars, sweets and
                 liquids, also refined foods or drugs.

Cracked skin = Possible disorders of spleen or pancreas.
   on feet

Becoming more aware of how to recognize and interpet
important changes in our bodies is one of the most impor-
tant steps in gaining control over our own personal health
*care. I hope that the information in **Simple Diagnostic Tests***
helps you to better understand how to approach the art of
self-diagnosis and I wish you and your loved ones the very
best of health.

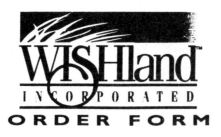

WISHland

INCORPORATED

ORDER FORM

Name _____ Phone _____

Address _____

City _____ State _____ Zip _____

Qty.	Item #	Description	Cost	Total
	W1500	Your Own Perfect Medicine by Martha Christy	$19.95	
	W1516	The Golden Fountain by Coen van der Kroon	15.95	
	W1501	The Water of Life by John Armstrong	11.95	
	W1900	Simple Diagnostic Tests You can Do At Home by Martha Christy	11.95	
	W1950	Healing Yourself with Homeopathy by Martha Christy	15.95	
	W1379	On The Track Of Water's Secret by H. Kronberger & S. Lattacher	14.95	
	W1902	Chemstrips Screening Test (10 Strips)	15.99	
	W1907	pH Monitoring Roll	11.95	
	W1505	PureaSkin Unscented Lotion	11.95	
	W1507	PureaSkin Unscented Cream	11.95	
	W1502	Scientific Validation of Urine Therapy by Martha Christy	11.00	
	W1503	You're in Good Health: 22 Testimonials of self-healing with urine therapy	11.00	
	W1504	Urine Therapy Introduction: Bruce Holmes Interviews Martha Christy	11.00	
	W1512	How To Fast On Urine Therapy	15.00	
	W1513	101 Ways To Use Urine Therapy	11.00	
	W1509	USP Grade Urea Crystals (1 lb.)	15.00	

Shipping & Handling
1 - 3 Items $ 4.00
4 + Items $ 8.00
10 + Items $10.00
Next Day Service Available.

Foreign Orders, ADD $25.00 to charges.

Arizona residents only - ADD 7.5% TAX

TOTAL AMOUNT ENCLOSED

Make checks payable to *Wishland, Inc.*
For Credit Card orders, call **1-800-559-2873**   ❑ Visa   ❑ MC   ❑ Discover   ❑ Am Ex

Acct. # _____Exp. Date _____

Signature_____Date _____

Send Order to: Wishland, Inc.,   Box 12172, Scottsdale, AZ 85267
(602) 922-8511   Fax: (602) 443-3386   To Order: 1-800-559-2873

Wishland Order Form

Item #	Description	Cost	Quantity
W1905	*Simple Diagnostic Tests You Can Do At Home* by Martha M. Christy	$12.95	
W1902	Chemstrips Multistix (10 ct.)	$14.99	
W1903	Chemstrips Multistix (100 ct.)	$95.00	
W1905	Sulkowitch Calcium Loss Test	$9.50	
W1907	pH Roll 4.5 – 7.5 (15' – approx. 3 month supply)	$11.95	
W1500	*Your Own Perfect Medicine* by Martha M. Christy	$19.95	
W1950	*Healing Yourself With Homeopathy* by Martha M. Christy	$15.95	
	Shipping and Handling: Shipping on all domestic orders over $35.00 is free. For orders under $35.00, please add $5.00 for shipping and handling. For foreign orders, please add an additional $25.00 for shipping and handling.		
	Arizona Residents Only: Please add 7% Sales Tax.		
	Total		

Please send your check (made payable to **Wishland, Inc.**) and completed order form to:

Wishland, Inc.
P.O. Box 12172
Scottsdale, AZ 85267
(602) 922-8511

Or call, toll-free: 1-800-559-2873

Or FAX us at: 1-602-443-3386